Doping's Nemesis

Doping's Nemesis

Arne Ljungqvist

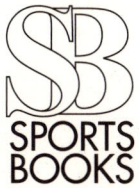

SPORTS
BOOKS

Published in Great Britain by
SportsBooks Limited
1 Evelyn Court
Malvern Road
Cheltenham
GL50 2JR

© 2008 Göran Lager & Ersatz
Published in the English Language April 2011

First Published as *Dopingjägaren*, 2008

A catalogue record for this book is available from
the British Library.

ISBN 9781899807 99 4

Printed and bound in England by TJ International.

Contents

Preface

THIS IS THE story of how I have tackled doping in the world of sport. I have dedicated more than half my adult life to this task. As such, this book is also the story of my life.

It didn't start out like that. It started off as an attempt simply to write the history of the fight against doping in sport. Time and again Swedish and international sports officials have encouraged me to write such a book. And time and again I have pushed that thought away. But eventually, I changed my mind. There did seem to be some who wanted this story to be told, and my perspective is unique.

I had been part of it all since the very beginning. And the others with me in that small group who started the anti-doping campaign forty years ago were no longer alive.

It is generally believed that the International Olympic Committee (IOC) has been responsible for driving the anti-doping campaign forward, but this is only partly true. The responsibility for managing international sport actually rests with the different international sports federations, and it was my place on the ruling Council of the IAAF – what is now known as the International Association of Athletics Federations – which was my platform for the work I did. It was there in the early 1970s that a true fight against the use of drugs in sport began.

I recruited leading scientists from the IOC's Medical Commission, Professors Arnold Beckett, from London, and Manfred Donike, from Cologne, to the IAAF's Medical Commission. Professor Beckett stood down in 1992, while Donike passed away in 1995. And the chairman of the IOC's Medical Commission, Prince Alexandre de Mérode, from Belgium, died in 2003. I am the only one left who can tell the whole story.

So assisted by a number of knowledgeable friends, I threw myself into the project. But it didn't work out. It wasn't possible to tell the story without also referring to my own background, my own life – both within and outside the world of sport. Everything was connected. So I put the project on hold.

I have always made a clear distinction between my public and my private life. I planned to carry on doing that. But people kept asking me questions. What had happened? Who did what? When will you write it all in a book?

So during the spring and summer of 2007, I picked up where I had left off, albeit with considerable reservations. While I have written hundreds of scientific articles, chapters in textbooks, and newspaper columns, I quickly realised that this wasn't a story I could tell on my own. So Lars Lundberg, a friend and a fellow sports official, made a series of taped interviews with me, interviews which were transcribed, edited and put into a written account by Göran Lager, a writer. Later, it was updated and translated into English with the financial support of the International Athletic Foundation

This is how the story of the campaign to tackle doping in world sport was written. It turned out to be a memoir, nonetheless. In spite of everything.

Arne Ljungqvist
Enebyberg, Sweden, February 2011

Chapter 1

Childhood

'OF COURSE I remember Per Albin Hansson. He was Sweden's Prime Minister before and during the Second World War. He lived near us, and he was well-known in our neighbourhood.

'I remember that he used to go for a walk along Ålstensgatan, wearing a hat and carrying a walking stick. He also used to take the tram. It was always the number twelve. It's still running. The Prime Minister taking the tram! It was as he was getting off the twelve one day that he collapsed and died. That was 1946.'

Ålsten in Bromma, was one of the first suburbs to spring up around Stockholm. Even at the start of the 1930s, Sweden's capital was surrounded by villages from where it was a long journey into the city.

Per Albin Hansson moved to Bromma in 1932, the year that he became Prime Minister. He moved into one of the houses along Ålstensgatan.

This was where the Swedish Welfare State was founded, the one Hansson spoke of in a parliamentary debate back in 1928. Nowadays, the functional, everyday houses along Ålstensgatan are among the most expensive in Stockholm. Their architecture and history makes them much in demand.

It was also here that Arne Ljungqvist was born in 1931, the year before Per Albin moved in. Ljungqvist's parents lived in Storskogsvägen, a street parallel to Ålstensgatan, which meant they lived close to architect Paul Hedqvist's famous terraced house, and were neighbours of the Prime Minister.

Along Storskogsvägen there were many fine houses. Developers had acquired the land for housing when it was open countryside. Those properties that weren't sold immediately were rented out to well-paid civil servants who wanted to move out from the heart of the city to the suburbs and be closer to nature. That's what Arne's parents, Gunnar and Solveig, did, not wanting to be tied down. As things turned out, they ended up staying in Ålsten.

In 1933, the family moved to Åsbacken, and three years later they moved into a large detached house at Tvärhandsgränd 5, which they bought at the end of the 1930s.

It wasn't just Per Albin who lived in the neighbourhood. Many of the senior figures in Sweden's Social Democratic Party moved to Bromma. They had children who would later go to school with Arne in Bromma. There, Arne's school friends included the children of Per Edvin Sköld, the Minister of Defence, who went on to become the Minister of Finance. They were known as the 'Sköld siblings'.

Other school friends included Lars and Hans Andersson, the sons of Karl Albert Andersson, the chairman of Stockholm City Council.

The villages of Ålsten, Nockeby, Äppelviken and Olovslund were like a large group of islands in Bromma. And until the bridge at Traneberg was opened in 1934, Bromma itself was something of an island. Until then, rural Bromma's only connection to the more industrialised Kungsholmen and the road through to Stockholm was just a slighty unstable pontoon.

Thus Bromma was not truly a part of Stockholm until they built the 580-metre-long Traneberg Bridge. The bridge, just like Per Albin's house on Ålstensgatan, was designed by Paul Hedqvist.

BEFORE THEY MOVED there, Arne Ljungqvist's parents had no obvious connection to Bromma. His father Gunnar was born in 1898 in Ockelbo, 200 kilometres north of Stockholm, where Arne's grandfather was a rural dean. Arne's mother, Solveig, was a provincial doctor's daughter from Söderköping, a coastal town about 150 kilometres south of Stockholm. Gunnar and Solveig met in Uppsala, where Gunnar was at university studying Law, Philosophy and Political Science.

'My father ended his studies prematurely with a bachelor's degree. He got a job as a telephone salesman, selling insurance, and this was the start of his career. He ended up being chief executive officer for what is now Trygg-Hansa, one of Sweden's major insurance companies.'

That's Gunnar Ljungqvist's career in a nutshell. The longer version tells of a string of companies, some that prospered, some that did not. It includes tales of double-dealing and bankruptcy, and of the scandal when the police arrested a number of senior executives in the world of finance.

Gunnar Ljungqvist, the young salesman, had been spotted by an executive at Skandia and headhunted. At that time, Skandia was the largest insurance company in the country, based at Skeppsbron, in central Stockholm. Things went well there for Gunnar, as he climbed the career ladder. Eventually, he was approached with an offer of another job from another Stockholm insurance firm, Städernas Försäkringsbolag. This was mutually owned by the company which was formed after the great fires of the nineteenth and early twentieth centuries which had reduced the forestry cities of Sundsvall, Härnösand and Umeå to ash.

The chief executive officer of Städernas Försäkringsbolag was Charlie Juhlin-Dannfelt. He was, for a time, also Stockholm city's finance commissioner, and so was very well-known throughout the city's financial and cultural circles. It was in his role as Stockholm's financial commissioner that he became involved in the Kreuger Crash, was charged and sentenced to jail.

'But my dad had at least been noticed by Charlie. Eventually, he succeeded Charlie as the CEO there. It's important to know – so that history is correct – that Städernas Försäkringsbolag was a very successful company during my father's time. When they started to expand they did so by first buying a company which was listed on the stockmarket but struggling: it was a maritime insurance company called Hansa.

'It was all about getting more customers and at the same time saving Hansa. It was like killing two birds with one stone.

'My father wanted to expand the company by offering life insurance. The company had only covered property and liability insurance, but then taken on maritime insurance through the purchase of Hansa. Now they bought a small life insurance company called Trygg. The company name now became Städernas-Trygg-Hansa, though they would drop Städernas from the title because it didn't work internationally.

'All this took place in the 1950s. The last thing my father did was to purchase the joint-stock limited company Separators' plot of land on Fleminggatan in Stockholm. Trygg-Hansa are still based there today. "I'm leaving it in good hands," he said. "My successor can develop the site." My father had a lot of foresight.'

While Gunnar was building his career, Arne's mother Solveig stayed at home with Arne and his three brothers. She had a maid to help her, as was common at the time. Solveig was five years younger than Gunnar, born in 1903.

'My mother never got any kind of university education after finishing school, unlike her other siblings. She had a younger brother and an even younger sister. The tradition was that the eldest child stayed home to "help on the farm", so to speak. My maternal grandparents had a large ramshackle house in Söderköping. They were a very social family, very active and knew a lot of people. My mother helped out like a maid at home when she was young.'

In Bromma, nearly every family lived in a spacious house, the children had a mother who was always at home and they often had a maid to help with the cleaning, making food and taking care of the children. 'It wasn't until my father died from a heart attack in 1968, just seventy years old, that my mother got a job at the Swedish International Development Co-operation Agency, although it was unpaid. She needed something to do to pass the time.'

It was the fate of her generation: women didn't make any contribution to their pension so they didn't receive a pension, and so were often left very poor towards the end of their lives. Gunnar, however, had left a pension that supported Solveig. She died, aged ninety-five, in 1998, when Arne was at the Olympic Games in Nagano.

LITTLE EIGHT-YEAR-OLD Arne was in Grade 3 at school when the Second World War broke out. Although Sweden remained neutral throughout the war, with neighbours Norway invaded by Germany and Finland by the Soviet Union, life in wartime Stockholm was constantly overshadowed by the threat of invasion.

'I went to school under the fear of war. Sure, it was more dangerous for those that were directly affected by the war, for children in our neighbouring countries, but the pressure we Swedes lived under has been underestimated.

'I remember how my mother sat there sewing identification tags into all our clothes in case war broke out. If it did, we were to be evacuated to Munsö by Lake Mälaren. The story of how Swedes lived under the threat of war has been forgotten.'

In 1940, Arne was aged nine and at primary school. 'We were a very similar circle of childhood friends. Even though it was a serious time we were allowed to behave like children.' In Ålsten, Arne and his friends spent their time competing to see who could run round the neighbourhood the quickest.

The streets Åsbacken, Brötvägen, Örnbogatan and Nyodlingsvägen made a square. Even today, they are sleepy streets lined with detached houses, but there was even less traffic back then. Together, the streets made a half a kilometre circuit, and the short stretch of Tvärhandsgränd, Arne's street, made a sprinting track of about forty metres.

Arne was the quickest runner. 'I wasn't just faster than the children the same age as me; I was also quicker than those who were a few years older. I was the fastest over the shorter sprinting track and the longer jaunt round the block. I wondered: "What the hell is this?"' He carried the burden of his parents' worries about the war – but he ran, ran really quickly, spurred on by his mates.

'It wasn't a question of *whether* Sweden would be forced to go to war, but *when*. My father received his call-up papers summonsing him to the Army in Närke in central Sweden in preparation for war. He stayed for several months, waiting. As an adult, I came to understand how strongly he had reacted to the First World War as a teenager, particularly the trench warfare on the Western Front where thousands of young soldiers were killed for just a few metres of land which were then lost the next day.

'And here he was having to go through it all again, only this time as an adult, responsible for his family and four small children.

'Gunnar had served in the military during the First War and now he was called up again. It was all happening again. My parents' generation went through psychological hell twice.'

The war was the main topic of conversation everywhere, whether at home, school or at work. No one could avoid seeing the political watershed: Nazi or not a Nazi.

Even in Sweden, and among Arne's schoolteachers, it was clear there were two groups: Nazis and anti-Nazis.

'Among us lads there was a negative attitude towards the Nazis. There was a feeling that it was they, the Germans, who had started the war. They were also jointly responsible for the First World War. I heard Hitler speak on the radio in our living room in Ålsten. He fired up both himself and the people. It was horrid. At the same time, there were young people's battalions that played war, while the real war was going on outside the country.'

The U30 – or *Ungdomslandstormen* – in Bromma was a kind of home guard for young lads, considered by some to have been right-wing and reactionary. Someone who didn't think this was Jan Myrdal, who has become a noted author and left-wing political commentator. Back then, like Arne, he was another lad from Bromma. He applied to U30 and was accepted.

'I was never attracted to it. I was too young. But my brother, who was two years older than me, got involved when he was fourteen. It was a kind of Hitler Youth, although with no Nazi propaganda.

'We did lots of sport. Children and teenagers especially did sport in their free time. It was an important way of switching off and playing – getting away from the fear and uncertainty of war. We even established a small athletics club in the area, The Ålsten athletics association, ÅIF. It was me and some of the other lads in the area including my elder brother. I was always the youngest and I can see now that it was in the ÅIF that my interest for sport was born.'

AN ATHLETICS CLUB needs a sports ground. Arne and his friends made do with a neighbour's garden. They badgered the nearby sports ground at Stora Mossen for equipment, built edges to their running track and put together basic long jump and pole vault pits. The official opening ceremony was full of pomp and circumstance, with their parents as the audience.

'There must have been forty onlookers at our opening competition. I still have the prize I won for the pole vault in my neighbour's backyard. It is a thimble-sized lead cup someone had found in a dumpster, awarded as a trophy. Someone had carved "ÅIF First Prize" on it, so it was serious.'

The events that day were even recorded on film, Arne's mother Solveig using a camera Gunnar had bought in Berlin in 1938.

In 1941, Arne started at Bromma Secondary School. Teaching physical education were Mr and Mrs Lindau, a well-known and very experienced couple. They soon noticed how talented Arne was.

'In 1943, I won all the events I entered at the school's sports: the 60 metres sprint, long jump and throwing a ball. I was then selected for the Stockholm district championships, where I also won all three events, as well as sprinting the final leg in our school team's winning relay team.

'To this day, I remember my winning results: 8.3 seconds for the 60 metres, 4.49 metres in the long jump and 65.5 metres for throwing the ball. It was a big thing and was covered with a big spread in the local Stockholm newspaper. It perhaps wasn't such a good thing for a twelve-year-old boy suddenly to be written about so much in the press. The principal at Bromma Secondary School rang my parents to tell them about my success, but said at the same time that we perhaps ought to tread a little cautiously.'

AT THAT TIME, Sweden had two major athletes: Gunder Hägg and Arne Andersson. For all the children that played sport in their spare time, they were role models. Arne remembers being at Stockholm's Olympic Stadium when Hägg made his breakthrough.

'It was 1940 and a gala meeting. There was to be an attempt on the world record for the 3,000 metres. The world record had been set by the Finn, Gunnar Höckert. He had won the 5000 metres at the Berlin Olympics in 1936, with Sweden's Henry Kälarne taking bronze.

'Kälarne's real family name was Jonsson but he had taken the name "Kälarne" from his home village. He had gone for the world record several times without success. He was going to make a new attempt, as Höckert had been killed in the Finnish Winter War, aged just twenty-five.

'I stood with my father and older brother in the Sofia stand and I remember looking out across the stadium and thinking to myself: "God, think what it would be like to compete here!" There were massive cheers when Henry Kälarne came in at 8 minutes and 9 seconds, slashing Höckert's world record by more than 5 seconds.

'But what I remember most of all was the man who finished second, who competed in black trousers and a yellow top with a big black "K" on his chest. His name was Gunder Hägg and he came from absolutely nowhere and also finished ahead of Höckert's old record. He was a complete unknown. It was amazing. And I was there to see it!'

Henry Kälarne came from Kälarne in Bräcke, in the northern province of Jämtland. Not quite next to it is Albacken, Hägg's home town.

Hägg would go on to be heralded by the American press as the world's greatest athlete and he was happy to refer to himself as 'Gunder the Wonder'. He was also destined to be banned from athletics for life, along with both Kälarne and Arne Andersson, for competing for money at a time when athletics, and the Olympics, were strictly amateur.

They had accepted money from organisers of athletics events for several years. As early as the beginning of the 1940s, Hägg was warned that he faced a ban, but he continued to accept money. When he was eventually banned, he was the world record-holder of all seven flat racing distances between 1500 metres and 5000 metres.

In the 1940s it was taken for granted that an amateur was an amateur. 'Gunder Hägg had a profession alongside athletics. He was a fireman, just like Henry Kälarne. They did jobs that gave them the opportunity to compete and train.

'It is very important to see this case of banning in relation to the rules that were in place at the time. The stipulation that athletes should be amateurs was upheld as late as the 1972 Munich Olympics. It was only when Avery Brundage left his post as president of the International Olympic Committee that year and Lord Killanin took over that the rules ceased to be so strict.

Childhood

'The major change came in 1980 when Juan Antonio Samaranch became president and, in turn, invited professional athletes to compete in the 1988 Olympics.'

YOUNG ARNE WANTED to carry on competing in athletics, although he didn't have any ambition to compete at the elite level – in fact, he had no idea what that involved. The only thing he knew was that he was talented. He knew this thanks to his results in the local competitions he had taken part in.

'I knew I was going to carry on with sport and thought it was a lot of fun. At the same time there were alternatives to athletics: like skiing and ski jumping, for example. There was a jumping hill close to Stora Mossen's sports ground. But that sport required winters with plenty of snow.'

Otherwise there was also handball, which Arne played indoors in the winter. Apart from handball, Arne wasn't interested in any other team sports: football didn't exist at all in his world. Football wasn't for the teenagers in Arne's part of Broma: that was for working class children.

In the summer there was always plenty of time for sport. Arne, however, had interests also outside sport. He was school champion in chess, and trained himself to become quite a good magician. He and a school friend would perform magic tricks on stage and at private parties.

In the 1930s and 1940s, Arne spent the summer holidays with his mother and siblings in the St Anna archipelago, close to Söderköping, Solveig's home town.

Among the upper-middle class in Bromma, it was common to go away to a summer house. Everyone did it. The Ljungqvists rented a summer cottage and had a sailing boat. Arne's father couldn't stay very long

– schoolchildren's summer holidays were considerably longer than a businessman's vacation.

It was during one of these long summer holidays that Arne had his confirmation service. It took place at Västerled Church, a modern, functional church built in 1932, designed by Birger Borgström. The church's building had been paid for, in part, by a collection raised in memory of Finn Malmgren, an Arctic explorer from Äppelviken who died on the polar ice in 1928.

It was Malmgren's mother who suggested making a collection in memory of her son. 'It didn't matter if you were religious or not. Getting confirmed was a kind of tradition.' Given that Arne's paternal grandfather was a country pastor meant that it was also part of the natural scheme of things in his family.

There were a lot of other things that were done by tradition and part of the 'natural scheme of things' in Arne's house. He was expected to do well at school, for example. Arne started elementary school a year earlier than his peers, taking his school leaver's certificate in five years. He spent one year extra at senior high school, thus keeping in line with his school mates.

'Most of my acquaintances graduated from senior high school. But there were also those who followed a more vocational path earlier. One of my earliest friends finished school early and became a photographer. I was actually quite lazy at studying, I think, and didn't really get down to serious work until the last couple of years of senior high school.

'Being involved in sport took up too much time, but I decided I wanted to carry on studying. So I had to be quite effective and study really hard towards the end. I graduated with good grades. However, I didn't have a sufficient combination of subjects to be able to go on to study medicine, so I ended up have to do extra maths whilst doing my military service.

'I think that school played an incredibly important part during these particular years, more so than before and in the years after. It was during the war. Society was more closed than it is now. The world was in chaos so you turned to what was closest to you: home, neighbours and school.'

Chapter 2

The High Jumper

'IT WAS DURING a school competition at the start of the 1940s that I saw a lad do the high jump. It was so beautiful. His name was Stig Frendin and he came from the city of Borlänge but was competing for Uppsala Enskilda Senior High School. He went on to compete for Sweden.

'When I practised at the sports ground at Stora Mossen, I tried to high jump using the scissors technique like he did. And I couldn't. There weren't any coaches, and no matter how I tried, the bar was always too high.

'Then suddenly I got it! I did several jumps in a row. I'd got the hang of it. I was perhaps twelve years old and the bar was set at 1.30 metres. Somehow I had chiselled together my own scissors technique. "Damn, this is really cool!" I thought.'

Arne had seen Gunder Hägg write athletics' history at Stockholm's Olympic Stadium. Arne Andersson, another great Swedish runner, was also one of his idols. It wasn't heroes like these that awoke Arne Ljungqvist's own interest in athletics, however. It was among the unassuming surroundings of the sports ground at Mossen, in school competitions, when competing against his peers, that Arne's fascination really developed.

Once he had got the hang of the high jump, it became Arne's main event. Success wasn't far around the corner either. As a thirteen-year-old he won the school championships in Bromma with a jump of 1.57m, and a year later, he improved his personal best to 1.63m. By the time he was fifteen, Arne even went on to compete at Stockholm Stadium in the Autumn School Athletics Games – the equivalent of today's Swedish national schools championships.

In 1946, the most promising athletes from Finland, Norway and Denmark were invited to participate. Arne, despite being the shortest of all the participants in the event in his under-16 age group, won with 1.71m.

'I can still remember who came second. It was a Dane called Malmkvist. He jumped 1.68. He came up to me afterwards and congratulated me, saying it had been a bloody good battle. It was great. The whole thing made the headlines. The sports journalists thought it was cool that a fifteen-year-old could jump so high – higher than himself.'

Arne continued doing other sports, too. During the winter he kept fit by playing handball for Äppelvikens SK. There weren't any indoor sports halls for athletics like there are today, which made track and field very much a summer-only sport. But there was a different attitude to training than there is today.

Arne enjoyed all the track and field events. 'I was a bit unusual because in addition to the technical events, I could also run.

'I ran, for example, the 1500 metres once in 4.22. I ran on my own, not competing against anyone at Stora

Mossen's track. Maybe I could have been a decathlete? There weren't many of those who could run the 1500m under 4min 30sec.'

THE FOLLOWING YEAR, Arne won the Autumn School Athletics again, this time with a jump of 1.80m. This put him among the junior elite. Åke Ödmark held the Swedish record with 2.00m. It was a major sensation that Arne, at just sixteen, had jumped so high.

'During the next year I had a knee injury which often hits adolescents: an inflammation of the tendon below the kneecap where it attaches to the shinbone. It's called *morbus Schlatter*, or what is also called Osgood-Schlatters Disease.

'It occurs in growing adolescents, particularly if they do a lot of sport. It heals, but it takes time and rest. You were often excused from gym for a term if you had *Schlatter*. So the year I was seventeen, I couldn't do very much. Still, I took part in the Autumn School Athletics Games and won again with 1.83m, a personal record.'

People began to notice this young high jumper, and they also saw that he was a good all-round athlete. When he was eighteen, he once again took part in the Autumn School Athletics Games. Over the years, it had become a big event, where to win one track or field event was a major triumph. That year, Arne won three: the high jump, the pole vault and the javelin. He was second in the discus.

Each year the Kungakannan – the King's Cup – was awarded to the best school that competed. Points were collected for each event. That year, Arne Ljungqvist single-handedly won the trophy for Bromma Secondary School. 'When I won the Kungakannan for Bromma Secondary School I set a personal best in high jump with 1.89. It was also a new Swedish schools record. Suddenly I had joined the elite.'

Among those who was now paying attention to this talented all-round athlete was Gösta 'Gösse' Holmér. Holmér had come fourth in the decathlon at the Stockholm Olympics in 1912. Now he was a national coach. 'Gösse Holmér said that he had never seen a high jumper like me before. And he also thought it might be worth me giving the decathlon a go. Sure, I think I could have been a good decathlete, but I didn't have any role models to inspire me.'

After he won the Kungakannan, Arne graduated senior high school and so entered compulsory military service. 'It was a complete waste of a year. I was in the Signals Regiment in Frösunda. I couldn't compete at all: I couldn't even train. It really was a waste. I couldn't compete until I was de-mobbed in 1951.

'Then I had to start all over again from scratch. I decided to concentrate on the high jump. I put everything into it!'

THAT ALSO MEANT that Arne would leave Stora Mossen behind him. When fifteen, he had joined the athletics club Westermalms IF, and it would be for them that he would broaden his competitive horizons.

'The first competition, a club match which Westermalm arranged in England, went dreadfully. I won, as it happens, but with something like 1.80, which was very mediocre. But my technique was improving and at a district championship in Stockholm, I cleared 1.91, another personal best.'

Arne was back among the Swedish high jump elite. A few weeks later, he won the gold medal at the Swedish junior championship.

There were a whole host of talented high jumpers at this time. One of them was Gösta 'Svängsta' Svensson. He was two years older than Arne and had jumped 2.00m. Another was Rune Reiz, who had cleared 2.00m a few years earlier. A third was Arne Åhman, who was really a triple jumper, the gold medal-winner at the 1948 Olympics, but he had high jumped 1.99m.

Arne went up against these three athletes for his first competition representing his country. It was 1951 and he had been selected as a reserve for the team that would compete in the annual meeting against Finland, the 'Finnkampen'.

'Even when I found out that I had been selected as a reserve, the management had put quotation marks around "reserve". It was pretty much understood that Åhman was only going to do the triple jump, so I would be the third high jumper.'

The event was a massive shock.

As the youngest, and as a reserve, Arne got to jump first. He started with 1.80, which he managed without problem. The bar was then raised to 1.85. Arne and all the other competitors cleared it on their first jump, except Rune Reiz, who crashed out.

'"Great," I thought. Not that Rune had crashed out, but that I wouldn't finish in last place. With the bar at 1.90, I failed at the first attempt. All three Finns cleared it on the first attempt, which the spectators loved. Svängsta cleared his first jump, and that silenced the crowd. I failed on my second attempt, much to the glee of the spectators.

'That made me so furious that I made my final jump out of pure anger – and cleared.'

The bar was raised to 1.93. Arne was first up – and sailed over! Another personal best. All three Finns stumbled at the first attempt, as did Svängsta. Suddenly Arne was leading the whole competition. The Finns failed at their second and then final attempts, crashing out. Svängsta managed to clear it at the second attempt and the bar was raised to 1.96 with just Arne and Svängsta left in the competition. Both failed to clear each of their three attempts, leaving Arne Ljungqvist as the victor.

The *reserve* had won!

THE SEASON CONTINUED in much the same vein. At every meet Arne competed in, he improved his personal best: from 1.93 to 1.94, to 1.96, and then 1.98. 'It was a late September evening in Uppsala. Dark and chilly. The organisers were forced to put an extra floodlight on near the high jump so I could see the bar. It was on 2.00 metres. And I cleared it – the fifth Swede in history!'

And Arne was the first Swedish junior to jump 2.00 metres. He was just twenty years old and suddenly looked like one of the country's biggest hopes ahead of the 1952 Olympics in Helsinki.

'My sensational victory at the Finnkampen also bagged me the honorary prize as the competition's most surprising winner. The prize took the form of a silver-plated beaten copper coffee kettle. Strangely enough, the handle on the lid is the Olympic rings! The reason for this is that the Finnish coffee company Paulig had donated a limited number of kettles like this one, that were to be awarded as honorary prizes during the 1940 Olympics in Helsinki, which never took place because of the war.

'The Finnish Sports Confederation decided to hand these Paulig kettles to specially deserving athletes during selected prestigious games in Finland after the war. The Finnkampen in Helsinki was one of them. I've no idea how many kettles like this are in existence, but there aren't many.

'It was quite amusing when my parents, many years later, attended a very exclusive dinner in Helsinki and my mother was placed at the table next to Mr Paulig. When she mentioned to Mr Paulig that she had one of his kettles, he answered something along the lines of: "I don't think so, my dear Mrs Ljungqvist. There aren't many of them in existence. But there are many people who think they have one."

'When my mother explained to her table guest the reason she had one of his kettles, he was overjoyed: he had found one of his kettles.

'I also have another very unusual prize at home: "the Kabom Trophy". In its day it was a very prestigious prize, established by the clothing manufacturers Oscar Molander in Alingsås in 1928. It is a forty-five centimetres high trophy made of pure silver with a lid, which was awarded to the best Swedish athlete at a number of international competitions and championships. It was awarded 114 times, until 1963. I got it after my high jump victory when Sweden beat Germany at Stockholm Stadium in the autumn of 1951. Many years later, in the middle of the 1990s, I visited the Sports Museum in Vänersborg on behalf of the Swedish Sports Confederation. In a display case there was a "Kabom Trophy". I mentioned to the guide Harald Jakobsson – the driving force behind the museum – that I had one just like it at home. Harald stiffened, turned pale and stuttered "wh-a-a-a-a-a-a-t?"

'It turned out that he had just published a small book on the history of the Kabom Trophy and about everyone that had received one, but he hadn't managed to find out who had got it in 1951. He went home and rewrote the book. I have both editions.'

A LOT HAS happened to the high jump since Arne was actively competing. With the advent of deep foam matting, athletes were able to be more adventurous in their landing styles and hence different jumping techniques have evolved. 'It's certainly the case with the majority of technical events that results tend to level out, until a new technique is developed. Then results improve again.

'The Fosbury Flop is perhaps one of the clearest examples of a technical innovation in an athletics event. Dick Fosbury won the 1968 Mexico City Olympics with a 2.24 metres jump with his "flop", turning his back to the bar in the final approach and going over backwards, landing on his back. Today it remains the dominant technique used by high jumpers.

'I met Dick Fosbury for the first time at the IAAF Gala in Monaco in 2007. He doesn't just know me through the International Association of Athletics Federations, but also as a high jumper who used the scissors technique. He also started out doing the scissors but told me that his biggest problem with the scissors was that he had trouble getting his bottom up over the bar.'

The flop is a variation of the scissors. Between them is the straddle technique, which was the predominant style high jumpers used in the years immediately after Arne's career. Straddle jumpers used the inner leg for the take-off, while the momentum of the outer leg is thrust up to lead the body face downwards over the bar – the opposite of the scissors and flop.

For scissors jumpers, the landing was a problem and it was part of the technique to try to land safely on your feet. The straddle, however, ushered in better landing mats than the original sandpits. To begin with, they made a mound of sawdust and then covered it to form a massive cushion. After that, foam mats were introduced and made thicker to ensure that the landing would be risk-free. It was this development which made Fosbury's new technique possible.

'When you did the scissors jump you had to manoeuvre yourself after you'd cleared the bar so you landed safely. Fosbury could forget about that. He discovered that the more parallel he was to the bar as he approached it and the more parallel he was as he cleared it, the easier it was to lift his bottom up over it. Suddenly, one day, he discovered that he was jumping with his back to the bar, headfirst. He perfected the technique and the "Fosbury Flop" was born. He increased his personal best by 20 centimetres or so.'

The surface on which they approach the jump is also different today. Arne jumped off cinders, a covering of finely ground coal, sand and tar, which was pressed down by the foot as the athlete jumped up, thus losing a large part of the kinetic energy. With today's modern, rubberised track surfaces, high jumpers today benefit considerably in terms of kinetic energy because the springy surface on which they jump has a trampoline-like effect.

ANOTHER DIFFERENCE IS the training. In Arne's time as a high jumper, training was almost non-existent and there was no such thing as a coach. I competed simply to get into shape. The same went for most of our elite as well as the happy amateurs. 'The only schedule that existed was the competition schedule: there wasn't much of an organised training schedule. It was like that during the entire time that I competed. A few did some training, but it wasn't anything like nowadays. Svängsta, I know, did a bit of training but he also worked at the Swedish Sports Confederation's grounds at Bosön. It never occurred to me that athletics should govern my life, in spite of the fact that I had got as far as competing in the Olympics.'

If Arne had been competing today he might also have amassed a fortune from athletics. But during his day, amateur rules stipulated that you could only receive payment in one form. The organisers of events paid out small amounts of prize money to the athletics federation's account. They, in turn, could then give the competitors some money in expenses, but it was little more than 'pocket money'. This was how Arne managed to earn enough to buy a radio-gramophone at the end of the 1952 season.

It all sounds rather quaint nowadays: no training schedule, no coaches, no prize money, no sponsorship money. And, most importantly, no doping. It wasn't until eight years after Arne had retired from competitive athletics that the world would witness the first doping incident at the Olympic Games.

'During my career in elite athletics, I never once heard about "banned substances". Even the word "doping" was completely unknown – at least, when it came to people and athletics. I know that horses and dogs were doped so they performed better in competitions, and that the military had given soldiers medication so that they were able to stay awake while on duty. But no one talked about doping humans at that time.

'As far as I was aware, it started during the 1960 Olympics, which was the first to be broadcast on TV. A Danish cyclist died right in front of the world's eyes after taking some kind of stimulant. Understandably, the IOC took immediate action. At the start of the 1950s, though, the whole idea of doping was unheard of, absurd.'

THE SPORTING HIGHLIGHT of 1952 was to be the Helsinki Olympics. Arne was to compete in Yrjö Lindegren's magnificent arena, which had originally been designed in 1934 to stage the Olympic Games in 1940, which were cancelled due to the Second World War.

Arne, by now twenty-one, was in good form. He had just won the classic 'Midsummer Games' in Gimo with a jump of 2.00m.

There, at his first Olympics, he would start the competition with a 1.90m opening height. But a small difference between the high jump of Arne's day and the present day was about to become of major significance for him.

There was a rule at that time that stated that athletes were only able to pace out their run-up before the competition. After that, you weren't allowed on the run-up until it was your turn to jump. A jumper today would laugh at this. In 1952 jumpers had their own different coloured foot-markers with which they marked out the run-up.

'I paced out my run-up and marked it. When I came to my first jump, I ran right into the bar. I didn't understand what had happened. It made me nervous, so I took it very carefully as I did my second jump because I realised how wrong I was. Full of the jitters, I just cleared 1.90.

'But it was the same for 1.95: I got a good lift-off but was too far from the bar so I hit it. My second attempt was much better; my body easily cleared the bar but I knocked it with my hand. On my third attempt, I did what I'd done on my first jump and crashed into the bar.'

Up in the stands, the Swedish supporters were trying to wave at him wildly. The sports medic Rolf 'Lammet' Ljungqvist – who Arne is still mistaken for even today even though 'Lammet' passed away a long time ago – had noticed what Arne hadn't. The Norwegian jumper Birger Leirud, with a personal best of 1.96m, had moved Arne's run-up marker thinking that it was his own. It was a complete catastrophe for Arne.

In those days, coaching from the stands was prohibited. Arne never realised what had happened and finished fifteenth. The gold medal was won by the American Walter Davis, and 'Svängsta', who Arne had beaten at both Gimo and the Olympic trials just a few weeks earlier, finished as the best-placed Swede in fourth with 1.98m.

There was no consolation for Arne when, just a few weeks after the Olympics, he beat the silver and bronze medallists, Ken Weisner, from the United States, and Telles da Conceicao from Brazil, at the same time as setting a personal best of 2.01m – just one centimetre from the Swedish record.

'When I found out what Birger Leirud had done moving the markers at the Olympics I was understandably upset and very disappointed. I'm certain I missed out on a medal because of what happened.'

AFTER THE DISAPPOINTMENT of the Olympics, Arne started to train more methodically. In the autumn of 1952, together with a number of leading athletes from the Swedish national team, he was involved in the setting up of Bromma IF, an athletics club.

'As well as myself, there was Lasse Ylander, Myggan Uddebom, Kacka Israelsson, Charla Johansson and Lennart Lind, to name a few. All of them lived in Bromma and belonged to the elite of Swedish track and field athletes. The idea was that we wouldn't be spread out among other athletics clubs, but united under one roof. Of course, I belonged to Westermalm IF, Ylander was in Tureberg IF, so it was quite weird always being together at Mossen.'

So Arne was back where it had all begun almost ten years before. Little did he imagine that his career as a high jumper would soon be over.

'What happened at the Olympics got me training over the winter ahead of the 1953 season because I knew how good I was. But I wasn't equipped to deal with all that hard training as it turned out. I didn't have the basic training necessary to really go for it big time.'

Arne started to feel some pain in the knee of his take-off leg. He was examined by, amongst others, 'Lammet'. 'No one could say exactly what the problem was. It just got worse and worse.'

In spite of the problem with his knee, and the fact that he was trying to rest, Arne accepted an invitation to take part in an event which would have major consequences for his career as an athlete.

'It was purely idiotic, but it's also a testament to how lightly we took athletics back then. It was a game.' The city of Stockholm was celebrating its 700th jubilee in the spring of 1953. The celebrations should actually have taken place the previous year, but they were delayed because of the Helsinki Olympics. The Stockholm Exhibition Centre down in Storängsbotten was involved in the celebrations and they organised a massive student carnival the like of which hadn't taken place in Stockholm for many years.

'We reintroduced a carnival which has continued to take place annually since then. Those of us involved in athletics in Bromma did something special. The carnival started out from Norra Real's school playground in central Stockholm. We appeared there, decked out as old athletes in cross-striped tops and silly trousers and with stacks of medals on our chest.

'Svängsta, Ylander, Erik Uddebom, Johansson and I were there. A few of them did a few short sprints, mucking about. Svängsta and I jumped over a bar that was balanced on the heads of two of the others.

'We did a high jump approximately every fiftieth metre the whole way from Norra Real through downtown

Stockholm to Nyloftet at Skansen (Stokholm's open air museum) where the whole thing finished with a party. We were doing the scissors over quite high jumps, landing quite hard on the concrete. Sure, we landed feet first, but it was hard.

'In the end, I did something like ninety jumps over 1.80 to 1.85 throughout the four-kilometre-long stretch. After that my knee was completely knackered. It never got better. The carnival was the final nail in the coffin. It was bloody awful!'

Arne went under the knife. At first they suspected it was an injury to the cruciate ligament. 'I was operated on by one of the leading experts on knee injuries at the time, a super specialist called Ivar Palmer. But not even he could see what the problem was. It wasn't so strange really as I was the first to get this injury which was unknown back then.

'Eighteen years later, in 1971 when I was at the Swedish championships in Umea in my capacity as a sports official, I learned that many high jumpers had been operated on for exactly this kind of injury: a kind of partial tear of the knee tendon. Today it's known as "jumper's knee" and is cured by routine treatment. But my athletics career was over at twenty-one years of age.

'If I had remained fit I certainly would not have retired from athletics. In spite of my medical studies, which I had already started, I would have certainly carried on jumping. I was so fixated on seeing how good I could get. I think I would also have gone for the decathlon ahead of the Melbourne Olympics in 1956. I wasn't really bad at any event except the shot put. It was really sad. There I was, just twenty-one and forced to give up my athletics career.'

It was one more important difference between athletics then and now: sports medical science.

Chapter 3

The Doctor

ARNE WAS JUST a boy when he decided that he wanted to be a doctor. What persuaded him was, partly, a number of people in his family and his neighbourhood were doctors: his maternal grandfather and his best friend's father. But there were also a number of incidents early in his life that influenced him.

'A number of my schoolmates died of polio and TB. That affected me. When we were about twelve, one of my friends in the scouts died after being treated with sulfa – an early antibacterial drug – when he had scarlet fever. Diseases like polio and scarlet fever were dangerous when I was a child. Nowadays, vaccines and antibiotics have changed that.'

In January 1952, Arne won a place to study at the Karolinska Institutet in Stockholm, noted as one of the world's leading medical schools, and the one which each year is responsible for choosing the winners of the Nobel prize in medicine or physiology.

He needed to take a few extra courses after graduating high school in order to be admitted. He had seven years of study ahead of him, or that was what it usually took, before he would be a qualified doctor.

First, though, he had to get used to the fact that his life as an elite sportsman was over. 'Of course I had to adapt my life after I stopped doing athletics. I was more like other people now.

'In 1957, I married my long-time girlfriend, Ulla, and together we had three children – Mats was born in 1957, Håkan in 1960 and Maria in 1964. A year before Maria was born, we moved to the house in Enebyberg, ten kilometres north of Stockholm, where I am still living.

'The children have all established themselves successfully, Mats, after graduating with a PhD in electronic engineering from Tokyo University, works as research co-ordinator within the European Union; Håkan is a businessman in a reputable food company following a university degree in economics at Uppsala University; and Maria, an economics graduate at Gothenburg University, works as the head of the asset management department of one of our largest banks.

'I now have seven grandchildren, one of whom has even followed in his grandfather's footsteps by studying medicine at King's College, London.'

ALONGSIDE HIS STUDIES, Arne became actively involved in the running of Bromma IF. Perhaps it was one way of adjusting to the fact that his own athletics career was over by supporting and getting behind others who were actively involved in athletics. 'People said that Bromma IF was just a flash in the pan, that the club would never amount to anything because only flashy elite athletes were involved. But we weren't worried. We had seen that there were masses of young people out there in Bromma who needed their own athletics club. So, sure, there was a certain amount of idealism behind what we were doing. That's what helped Bromma IF survive, in spite of all the prophets of doom. And the club is still one of the leading athletics clubs in Stockholm.'

EVEN DURING HIS time as a student at Karolinska, Arne made an important choice in terms of the direction his medical career would take. 'There were a number of lower recruitment paths aimed at enticing students into future careers in research. You could start out as a research assistant at a department. In 1957 I was offered a post as an assistant at the department of pathology at Karolinska. I thought it sounded interesting. I would get to see diseases in the real world, while other departments with assistant posts were more geared toward theory.

'The subject "pathology" can perhaps be best described as "the theory of illness", and it offered me a more practical exposure to disease. I would get the opportunity to synthesise all the theoretical knowledge I had gained from anatomy, histology, physiology and chemistry and apply it to actual patient cases. I thought it sounded exciting, so I accepted the offer.'

Pathology would thus become Arne's area of expertise, but only after he had completed his medical studies and gained practical experience within different fields. Shortly after he graduated, at the start of the 1960s, he worked for a number of years as a paediatric surgeon at Crown Princess Lovisa's Children's Hospital, which at that time was the largest children's hospital in Stockholm. He often returns to the subject of a dreadful tragedy that occurred there and was paramount in shaping his view of pathology.

'One day a ten-year-old girl came in. She had sprained her ankle while playing with her friends, just skipping. It was a trivial and common injury. When children like that come in and are in pain and have trouble putting weight on the foot, the best thing to do is have the ankle joints on both legs X-rayed. It's easier to compare them in order to see whether the sprain has injured the epiphysis, the growth zone which is just next to the joint in growing children. An injury like this is called epiphysiolysis, and must be treated like a fracture in order to prevent future problems.

'It can be quite difficult to see if it is epiphysiolysis or not. In this particular case, the radiologist didn't see anything wrong with the girl's sprained ankle. However, there was something not right with the uninjured ankle. At first glance it looked like an inflammation just above the growth zone. Despite the girl not having any symptoms apart from a sprained ankle, the discovery was so alarming that she was put under the knife so they could take a biopsy from the inflamed area and examine it under a microscope. I was then asked to take the sample to the pathology department at Karolinska because there was no pathology unit at Princess Lovisa's.

'Together with an older colleague at Karolinska, I examined the specimen under the microscope. Before I had a chance to say anything he exclaimed: "For goodness sake, this is cancer!"

'It was what is called an osteosarcoma. The girl had come in because she had sprained one of her ankles, but under the microscope the specialist could see that she had cancer in her other ankle.

'She was forced to have her leg amputated just below the knee joint. I remember I saw her once, cycling with her one leg a year or so later. But the osteosarcoma came back and I heard she didn't survive. It is common that secondary tumours occur with osteosarcoma and in those days there was no cure for that type of tumour. The only chance for survival was to operate, as we did.'

After his time at Crown Princess Lovisa's Children's Hospital, Arne returned to Karolinska. The case of the girl with the skipping rope and other practical work had shown Arne the significance of pathology. So after having worked for a year in intensive care, he finally decided to specialise in pathology.

The girl with the skipping rope is also an eloquent example of how cancer treatment has developed since Arne was a young doctor at Lovisa's Children's Hospital. Then, being diagnosed with cancer was like being handed a death sentence. 'Today we know that cancer isn't just one disease: it's found in many variations and each has its own prognosis and treatment. Just as we've improved how we diagnose things, and learned how to better differentiate between different forms of cancer, developing new targeted methods of treatment for the different subtypes of the disease, we have many different ways of treating patients successfully today.

'We count on fifty per cent of all cancers being curable nowadays.'

There are many examples of this. Testicular cancer in boys, which was lethal when Arne studied medicine, is one example. Today most cases are cured. The same goes for childhood leukaemia. Those children that were admitted to Lovisa's suffering from leukaemia during Arne's time as an assistant physician at the end of the 1950s and beginning of the 1960s were as good as living under a death sentence – at least ninety-five per cent of all cases proved fatal.

'It was one of the worst things you could experience: really sick children with a hopeless prognosis. It was really tough to deal with, even though you were expected to. Nowadays, childhood leukaemia is ninety-five per cent curable.'

A third cancer which in those days was fatal is a particular form of kidney cancer that affects children called Wilms' tumour. 'A young relative of mine died aged three or four from that cancer at the end of the 1950s. Doctors would probably have cured him today.'

Much work, of course, still remains to be done. Even in the 1950s people spoke about finding a vaccine for different forms of cancer. Nothing like that has been found yet. There remain forms of cancer which are extremely difficult to treat. One of these cancers is pancreatic cancer, which only gives symptoms very late and is very hard to diagnose in time to treat. Another is lung cancer.

'The number of sufferers from lung cancer has perhaps declined because the number of smokers has gone down, but cancer takes a long time to develop so those who are being hit now are often those who previously smoked a lot. When I was young many of the lads smoked but very few women. Between the 1960s and the 1980s it was the other way around. We're seeing the effects today: there are more women who are dying of lung cancer.'

Overall, however, there has been an enormous development. 'During my years as chairman of *Cancerfonden* (the Swedish Cancer Society) between 1992 and 2001 I was able to follow cancer research quite closely. It is the Swedish Cancer Society that gives financial support to cancer research and it is there that the combined expertise in the area is located. Donations that stream in are passed on to researchers. During the mid-1990s we were handing out between two and three hundred million Swedish kronor each year, equal to about US$30–40 million, making it the largest charity in Sweden. Today the figure raised each year is about $50 million. Thanks to the Society, cancer research in Sweden is still extremely strong. Because we also have a lot of money we attract leading researchers to Sweden.'

One of these researchers is Arne himself. 'As a pathologist, and later head of pathology at Karolinska, I have had the privilege of witnessing the development of different methods. A large part of my everyday work as a pathologist was taken up with diagnosing cancer. I did a lot of work under the microscope and running other tests to ascertain whether patients had cancer or not.'

The majority of a pathologist's routine work centres on diagnosing the illnesses of living people. It is about trying to determine whether the disease is malignant or not, and identifying exactly what it is. Sophisticated analytical methods are the basis of the work. One of these is cell analysis, also known as cytopathology, which is undertaken to ascertain the type of tumour.

'We're talking about Needle Aspiration Biopsy and Exfoliative Cytology. Needle Aspiration Biopsy means when a needle is attached to a syringe and is used to pull out cells from the suspected tumour. These are then studied under the microscope. These tests allow you to see whether it is cancerous or pre-cancerous by studying the appearance of different structural features which we call atypical. Needle Aspiration Biopsy is a wonderful diagnostic tool. After just a pin-prick a patient can be told almost immediately what the matter is, and receive the appropriate treatment.

'Exfoliative Cytology was initially developed to diagnose cancer of the cervix of the uterus, one of the most serious forms of cancer that hits young women. The method involves scraping cells from the mucus membrane of the cervix on to a microscope slide. The cells are then stained and analysed under the microscope. Diagnosing cancer of the cervix or pre-cancerous lesions early can save lives. Exfoliative Cytology enables us to routinely control patients. Today Sweden is a world leader when it comes to far-reaching preventative medicine for young women. It is rare nowadays that someone dies because of this form of cancer.

'To give an overview of how medical science has developed during our age is almost impossible. So much has happened just since I became a doctor. Antibiotics had been discovered before I even started studying. That was an incredible piece of progress which allowed many serious infectious diseases to be treated, particularly those that affected and killed children. The discovery of penicillin considerably reduced the incidence of child mortality.'

Transplantation procedures have also made incredible progress, particularly in terms of the anti-rejection medication that has been developed. The first kidney transplant in Sweden took place in 1964, just a few years after Arne qualified as a doctor. The doctor in charge of the surgery was a professor at the Karolinska Institutet, Curt Franksson. 'And later on an old childhood friend of mine, Göran William-Olsson, or "Jörpa" as we called him, carried out the first heart transplantation in Sweden in Gothenburg in 1984.'

A THIRD MAJOR advance in medicine is genetics. When Arne began studying to be a doctor, genetics did not have any significant clinical application. Today the complete genetic make-up of man is documented: this means that there is every chance of dealing with both hereditary diseases and diseases that occur as the consequence of external factors that have affected the genes.

Theoretically defective genes can be exchanged for healthy ones, and new genetic material can be added to patients who need it. Researchers are working to make this kind of gene transfer possible in practice, and some of them have succeeded. This approach is called gene therapy. It is opening up new fields of possible treatment, but also has the risk of being abused.

'There is a risk that genes will simply be swapped in order to develop new qualities and that in that way, individuals with tailor-made characteristics will be cultivated. An East German-like regime would be able to abuse research achievements in such a way. It's precisely this that is of concern to those of us working within athletics: we're worried that gene technology could be misused to create especially talented athletes with characteristics tailored to suit particular fields of sport. This is known as "gene doping".

'The threat exists already today and could be a reality tomorrow. I have therefore taken the initiative of acquiring knowledge about the possibilities to hinder such abuse. I would also dare to claim that we have the expertise necessary to lay out a genuine strategy and we work intensively to develop the tools needed for testing in order to reveal whether a human has been exposed to gene manipulation.'

This work is widely supported by geneticists who are adamant that the technique should not be misused and that gene therapy as a science should not come into disrepute.

ARNE'S CAREER AS an elite athlete had finished almost before it had begun. When Arne thought that his sporting career was behind him forever, medicine replaced athletics. Yet a notable career combining the two aspects of his life was awaiting him.

Arne completed his doctoral thesis in 1963, just four years after qualifying as a doctor. Shortly thereafter he became a senior lecturer. Towards the end of the 1960s, he was appointed assistant professor, which became a full professorship in 1979. In 1972, twenty years after the Helsinki Olympics, he became the vice-dean of the medical faculty at the Karolinska Institutet, the second most senior post among the professors of the medical faculty, responsible for the institute's medical training. He was only forty-one years old.

Five years later he became the vice deputy chancellor of the Karolinska Institutet, a post he held until 1983.

Arne's decision to study medicine and later complete his doctorate in pathology wasn't an end in itself. It was the day-to-day reality of his job and his research which gave him satisfaction.

'I've enjoyed working in research connected to health care. The Department of Pathology engages in research on a daily basis in the sense that you diagnose patients, applying research-like methods and procedures. The duties also include ascertaining the cause of death, and I regard the profession as a form of "quality control" of the healthcare system. Once we have ascertained the cause of death we can compare the clinical observations made during a patient's lifetime with our findings. The knowledge we gain by this is incredibly valuable and helps the development of future progress.'

Arne was relatively young – thirty-two – when he completed his doctoral thesis. PhDs his age were usually those that had either dropped out of the undergraduate studies or made a temporary pause because they had become fascinated with a very specialised topic. Arne was both a qualified medical doctor and a PhD. 'It was pretty advanced. I had become interested in kidneys, but in the light of the methods that exist today my thesis isn't really that technically significant, but it was back then. It dealt with the blood supply of the kidney. I studied the distribution and behaviour of the most minute blood-carrying vessels in the normal and diseased kidney.

'To study this I used a technique which made it possible to X-ray the blood supply of the kidney. I injected barium sulphate contrast to be able to follow minutely how the arteries branched into arterioles and capillaries. Then I constructed a new microscope which could show the pictures stereoscopically. In this way I created a three-dimensional picture. This was innovative within the context of the study.'

No matter how far Arne's new career path led him away from athletics, he still carried his experience with him. 'I certainly worked hard. This is something I've always done. I think I learned how to be single-minded through sport – a kind of self-discipline that has benefited me my entire life. Many times people have wondered how the hell I managed everything: my answer is that I learned a lot from sport.

'I've learned two things in particular: first, ever since I was young I have understood how important it is to be well-organised. Secondly, I understood from a young age how important it is to delegate to competent people who are working around you. They also then feel that they have to take their responsibility, which in turn creates a sense of job satisfaction. I have always striven to create teams that work well together.

'I have seen so many bosses who can't delegate. This in turn makes all their co-workers unhappy. I have trouble understanding this, for no other reason than self-preservation: you have to be able to delegate to get some time for yourself.'

When Arne became assistant professor at the end of the 1960s, the post was a tenured state-appointed professorship. It gave him a guaranteed salary, a team of co-workers, quite often a secretary and a lab assistant as well as a research grant. Of those appointed to a professorship in the old Swedish system –and this included Arne – there are many who feel that the term 'professor' is banded about too easily nowadays. Any college of higher education today can appoint someone as 'professor'.

'When I applied for my chair, there were three candidates. We were all highly qualified MDs with PhDs and our qualifications were scrutinised and evaluated by three professors from different universities. In other words, it was a competition, and a professorship was much coveted. Today, they are handed out as titles without any further resources.'

Back then it was also the state that determined which areas of research should be awarded a professorship and given guaranteed research funding. 'In this way research could be steered to areas that were of national importance.'

THE DEMANDS OF Arne's medical career left him little time for anything else. 'Athletics was a closed chapter for me for a long time. I had gradually withdrawn from all involvement in Bromma IF. I simply didn't have any spare time and, honestly, I wasn't even that interested in following sport as there were too many other things that caught my interest.

'Then in the 1970s, my background in athletics and medicine came together. I usually say that it was my toughest decade.'

One day in 1971, the telephone rang at Arne's home. It was Karl-Axel Torége, the chairman of the Swedish athletics association's nomination committee. 'He told me that one of the members had walked out on the board in a fit of anger after one or two decisions he had been unhappy about. They now needed someone to replace him. What's more, the then president of the association, Matts Carlgren – one of the country's leading industrialists and accordingly a very busy man – was also rumoured to be on the verge of resigning.

'I was told during our first conversation that I was being considered for the post of president for the Swedish athletics association. *What*? Of course, I was flattered to be thought of as the leading figure in Swedish athletics, but I was very surprised.

'But I suppose I wanted to see how things were today so I said "Yes" to Karl-Axel Torége.'

Arne was duly elected to the board in 1971 with a view to taking over the leadership in 1973.

'When I took over the leadership, I discovered that elite athletes were talking about completely different things than we did during my time, twenty years earlier. Back then we talked about all sorts of things in life, about how we lived, how we ate, and how much fun we had.

'Now all they were talking about was which pills to take to become a better athlete. I approached this as a qualified doctor and I wondered what the hell they were talking about! Pills to be a better athlete?

'I felt that I had landed in a very alien environment so I decided to try to find out more about what elite Swedish athletes were busying themselves with before I took any action.'

Arne compiled a questionnaire which he sent out to all the top-ten male athletes in 1972. It turned out that the pills Arne had heard the athletes talking about were anabolic steroids. 'I asked myself what the hell they were doing! Anabolic steroids were medication developed to strengthen a withering body. They were given to patients in the final stages of cancer or with severe chronic inflammations, TB or other similar diseases, to build up a body which was deteriorating. They were meant to give patients a chance.

'Anabolic steroids increase the protein synthesis in the body, and thus strengthen the tissue, muscles, bone mass and inner organs in general. But if you start using these medicines on people that don't need them, I knew that this could have completely different results. It is completely absurd to use anabolic steroids to give a healthy person additional strength. It's like giving insulin to a non-diabetic. The effects can be disastrous and completely unpredictable. Once again I asked myself what the hell Swedish athletes were doing.'

The findings of the questionnaire were published in the *British Journal of Sports Medicine* and it caused a sensation. Nothing like this study had ever been done before and it is still cited today in current scientific articles on sports and anabolic steroids.

One-third of those who were approached did not fill in the questionnaire as they did not trust that they could be guaranteed full anonymity. Almost one-third of those who answered had tried, or were still taking, anabolic steroids.

It is easy to assume that many of those who avoided answering the questionnaire were also using this kind of medication. That would mean that between one-third and a half – perhaps even more – of all Sweden's elite athletes were using anabolic steroids in 1972.

'I felt that I was at a crossroads and declared that I could not lead an organisation where such behaviour was going on. It went against everything that I had learned or taught during my medical career.

'I thought I could either kiss goodbye to my involvement in the whole set-up, or I could try to do something about it. I remember that I had a conversation with the vice-chancellor of the Karolinska Institutet, Sune Bergström, who later won the Nobel Prize for Medicine. I remember that Sune said: "Arne, you have to do what you can to put a stop to this. You have what is needed. You have a background as an athlete, but also as a physician and scientist. These are our young people, who are doing something really dangerous. We must, as professors and researchers, be prepared to go out into society and contribute to its sound development."'

In other words, Arne had the full support of the Karolinska Institutet.

But the story could have turned out quite differently.

ARNE WAS ALSO on the Karolinska Institutet's faculty committee. He would soon become vice-dean, responsible for the institute's medical programme. But this was in an era when the shockwaves of the Paris riots of 1968 were still being felt around Europe. One effect was that Sweden's Ministry of Education and Science, in typical Swedish fashion, instigated an inquiry to assess how universities were organised and governed. It was called the 'U 68'. After nine years, the inquiry's findings were presented under the name 'H 77'.

A suggestion that was made towards the end of the inquiry's report was that all the study programmes run by the universities and university colleges in Stockholm should be grouped together under the jurisdiction of a single 'Stockholm University College'. In keeping with 1968-style ideology, the term 'university' was considered too formal a term, implying some kind of elitism. So instead, it was to be called 'University College'. And it was to be massive and all-encompassing. There were to be no departments that stuck out.

The Karolinska Institutet was, thus, to fall under its jurisdiction and be known as 'The Medical Programme at Stockholm University College'. The Royal Institute of Technology (KTH) would also vanish and be known as 'The Engineering Programme at Stockholm University College'.

'I remember that Sune Bergström, our vice-chancellor, was astounded and confused. So was the dean as well as the majority of the faculty. The vice-chancellor, dean and I were commissioned to make a so-called personal courtesy call on the education minister to draw attention to how ludicrous it was for Sweden to dispense with such world famous research institutions such as the Karolinska Institutet and KTH.

'The education minister in the new, non-Socialist government which came to power in 1976 was Jan-Erik Wikström. I remember our "courtesy call" very clearly, along with the education minister's comments.

'"Gentlemen," he said. "It's not possible. It has already been agreed upon by the Center Party (the largest non-socialist party, which the prime minister belonged to) and the Social Democrats (the largest opposition party)." So it really looked hopeless.

'But then along came Alfred Nobel's will to save us. It turned out that the regulations that would come into force if a combined University College was formed were irreconcilable with the stipulations outlined in Nobel's will. The new University College would not be able to award the Nobel Prize for Medicine, and nor would any other authority. So it was this that forced the politicians to reconsider.

'It's funny that Alfred Nobel contributed to me being able to combat doping for all these years. I don't think I would have been able to count on any support from the planned large-scale University College.'

Chapter 4

Steroids: The First Battle

IN THE WORLD of sport that Arne returned to in the early 1970s, drugs were part of everyday life.

People had only just begun to realise that they were a problem. There was almost no information about how widespread drug use was, no regulations, no functioning drug tests. Taking anabolic steroids wasn't even against the rules. 'But Matts Carlgren was one person who believed that drugs was a major battle for athletics. And with my medical training I understood that the use of steroids was completely ludicrous. Yet even though they had dangerous side effects, it was completely legal to take them.'

There was already a medical committee within the International Olympic Committee. It was formed in 1961, following the death of the Danish cyclist Knud Jensen, during the road race at the 1960 Rome Olympics. Rome was the first Olympic Games to be broadcast live internationally, the first 'TV Olympics'. When Jensen collapsed, he did so in the living room of millions of viewers. They wanted an answer. Why had this happened?

The initial post mortem reported that Jensen's death was caused by heatstroke. But it turned out that Jensen had performance enhancing substances in his body. He, like his team mates, had been given them by his coach to combat fatigue and improve his performance. The substance was said to be amphetamine, which today is classed as a narcotic. Ultimately, it was a combination of the stimulant and the heat and exertion that cost Jensen his life, while his team mates, utterly exhausted and in a serious condition, needed to seek medical attention after the race.

THE HISTORY OF drugs in sport is as long as the history of sport itself. Long before the term 'doping' was used, competing athletes had experimented with something or other, unconcerned that they were cheating, and often without thought that it could be dangerous.

Barrie Houlihan, a political scientist at the Institute of Sport and Leisure Policy at Loughborough University, has studied sport from a sociological perspective. Houlihan claims there is evidence to suggest that performance enhancing substances were used by the ancient Greeks. Athletes ate figs riddled with a fungus which was said to improve their performance.

The Romans gave their gladiators substances to combat fatigue after long sword fights.

And when the amphetamine that cost Jensen his life was finally classed as a narcotic in Sweden in 1974, athletes instead started to use ephedrine – another performance-enhancing substance. This was made from the ephedra plants, known as *ma huang* in China, whose medical properties are mentioned in 5,000-year-old Chinese documents.

At the end of the nineteenth century, when organised sport began to resemble the form that we know today, substances such as nitroglycerine, alcohol in the form of schnapps and cognac, strychnine and opium, caffeine, heroin and cocaine, were all used, often mixed into 'cocktails'.

It was also around this time that the term 'doping' was first used. The first example of the word being formerly defined, according to Björn Sandahl at Södertörn University in Stockholm, is in an English dictionary in 1889, as: as 'a morphine-like substance which is used with the purpose of worsening a horse's performance within a racing context' – ironically, therefore, as a performance-inhibiting substance.

It was not long, however, before people started giving their horses substances to *enhance* their performance on the race track. This practice was banned in 1910, and doping tests in the world of horse racing were introduced the same year.

However, doping would not be banned or tested for within human sport for many years. Jensen's high-profile death, nevertheless, put the world of cycling under scrutiny for doping: regulations and anti-doping tests were set in place. Even today, however, one top cyclist after another is found to have taken drugs.

It was not long before doping began to be discussed within other sports, too. The Football Association in England carried out testing as early as the 1966 World Cup, and after this, some crounties introduced anti-doping rules.

'But at the beginning of the 1970s, the international sports federations were very passive. It was only at the Olympic Games that doping tests were performed.

'The first thing that I reacted against was that fully fit international athletes were being allowed to take anabolic steroids. There was so little information about what side-effects they could have and, of course, it was impossible to run tests on humans to see what effect they had. There weren't any scientific studies on what side-effects athletes taking anabolic steroids might experience, or how their performance might be enhanced.

'What we scientists call "reliable experience" told us that the very high doses taken by athletes could prove dangerous, but when, even as recently as 1982, we announced this in the *Journal of the Swedish Medical Association*, we were ridiculed.

'No athlete wanted to hear what we were saying about dangerous side-effects. They were convinced that steroids enhanced their performance.'

Athletes have always tried to improve their performance by diet. In modern times it has created a multi-billion-dollar global industry which produces vitamins and all sorts of supplements sold in the form of tablets or beverages. This has conditioned athletes to see supplements as something completely 'natural' and 'safe' when taken at the right dose. And there, out on the market alongside the other supplements, were steroids.

Steroids had been available since the 1930s when they were first produced. Anabolic steroids are a synthetic variation of the hormone testosterone. Among the well-known side-effects is a significantly increased level of aggression. Steroids replaced amphetamines as the aggression-enhancing substance given to soldiers during wartime. There are still examples today of people who have committed violent crime, even murder, with synthetic steroids in their body.

'One athlete in the national team – it doesn't matter who – called me one day at the start of the 1970s and told me that he had been out for a few beers with a friend when things had got out of control. He had become aggressive and when the police were called he was arrested and placed in a cell. He was charged with assault.

'He wondered whether the fact that he took steroids and had had a couple of beers could explain his behaviour. I told him that this could well be the case. It was a clear example of a bout of aggression brought on by a combination of alcohol and steroids.

'Today the link between steroids, alcohol and unprovoked acts of violence is widely recognised.'

IT WAS IN the Eastern bloc that athletes were first given access to amphetamines and testosterone in a systematic manner, and to such a degree that it influenced results in sporting events. In the late 1950s and early 1960s, athletes from the Soviet Union and other Eastern bloc countries began to perform significantly better than earlier, sometimes even better than their "comrades" from the West. There was drug-use among athletes in the West, but not in an organised or state-funded system.

To measure up with their competitors from the East, individual athletes and coaches in the West contacted doctors, some of whom freely made prescriptions available. Pharmacies became some kind of indispensible smorgasbord for athletes. A good diet, enough sleep, training and technique just wasn't enough to compete any longer. That little extra chemical kick had become indispensable.

As president of the Swedish athletics association, Arne made his first trip in 1973, along with the Swedish athletics team, to an international competition in Norway. He was struck by how good the Swedes had become in all the throwing events.

The results in shot put that day were so good that it would have placed all three participating Swedes among the top six in the Sydney Olympic Games final twenty-seven years later.

'I don't want to accuse all of them of doping, but one of them, Ricky Bruch, has at least admitted it publicly. He was world record-holder in discus and bronze medal-winner in the Munich Olympic Games in 1972.

'You just have to remember that it wasn't illegal to take steroids back then. It wasn't even regarded as immoral, more like a healthy supplement. After my questionnaire I knew that performance-enhancing substances were widely used by Swedish athletes. I realised that I needed to "put my own house in order" before tackling the problem on an international scale. So we introduced regulations and drug tests at competitions in Sweden as an initial attempt to stop the problem. Those athletes that were taking pills didn't have a clue what they were actually doing; they still thought they were popping performance-enhancing vitamins into themselves, so I can understand those who approached me, upset and angry. I'm not accusing them. The new rules and drug tests were not popular amongst athletes and one of the most vocal was Ricky Bruch.'

The conflict reached a climax in 1977. Sweden was to compete against East Germany and the national team was taken by bus down from Berlin airport to Halle, where the competition was to take place. On the coach, the team ganged up to form a veritable revolt, led by Bruch. They demanded Arne Ljungqvist's resignation in writing on account of his involvement in anti-doping. The letter was signed by practically all the athletes. Arne was really under pressure.

'I was furious. I summoned them to a meeting that evening where I attempted to explain why I was acting against doping. I don't think that everyone bought my explanation, but I think I managed to persuade the majority of them. I also explained that I had no intention of resigning.

'Ricky Bruch would later go on to become a supporter in the fight against doping, and also a good friend. He wasn't just an exceptionally talented athlete, he was also a very special person. He had the capacity to capture the media's interest, for both good and bad, when it came to him both as a person and an athlete. He did one spectacular thing after the other.

'I remember that I once complained to the then president of the Swedish skiing association: skiing had Ingemar Stenmark, a calm and well-liked man as its leading star. I had to deal with Ricky Bruch. It wasn't fair!'

Arne didn't resign in Halle. Instead the incident strengthened his determination to tackle doping. Outwardly, he appeared like calmness itself. But when Sweden's national team, headed by Ricky Bruch, demands the resignation of the head of the national association, it makes headlines. The events in Halle set off the first media campaign against Arne. Both he and his family had to get used to journalists ringing in the middle of the night, asking for comments or trying to dig up all conceivable facts about him.

'It was my first experience of being publicly examined, but I certainly knew what I was doing and was young and strong back then. I took the commotion as a clear indication that something really seriously needed to be done. I understood that I wouldn't be able to do anything about doping internationally until I had dealt with it in Sweden first. I was sure that it was necessary, even if it meant costing us results for a generation of elite athletes.'

WITHOUT PERFORMANCE-ENHANCING drugs, Swedish athletes in international competitions would be beaten before they had even started. Swedish athletics needed a long-term goal.

'The most important thing was to start spreading information and educate the upcoming generation of elite Swedish athletes. To turn to the young people. I had become a member of *Riksidrottsstyrelsen* – the board of the Swedish Sports Confederation – in 1975 and was the only one there with a medical background. But I got the board to go along with me and we started developing strategies to combat doping. It was one thing trying to get the information to users, another to try to get at the suppliers.'

It was just as important to map out where the drugs were coming from as it was to make Swedish athletes aware of the dangers of doping. In Sweden there was only one legal way of getting steroids, and that was on prescription. There was a theory then that they were being prescribed by unscrupulous doctors.

A joint investigation was undertaken with the Swedish state pharmacy and the National Swedish Board of Health and Welfare to find doctors who had a suspicious pattern of prescribing drugs. The results were not as had been suspected. Of course, some doctors were found prescribing steroids. However, Arne's questionnaire had suggested that almost half of the competing elite athletes took steroids, so way more drugs were being used than prescribed by these few doctors.

It meant that Arne and the officials had to rethink. Substances were evidently being smuggled into Sweden from abroad. The problem of doping could clearly not be resolved on a purely national level.

It was also critical that some form of drug testing programme should be introduced. The first time tests were carried out to detect anabolic steroids in athletics was at the 1974 European Championships in Rome.

Arne had become a member of what was then called the International Amateur Athletics Federation (later changed to the International Association of Athletics Federations), or IAAF, medical committee in 1972. The chairman of the committee, Max Danz, made him responsible for the IAAF's anti-doping programme. Danz was an older doctor in private practice in Germany and had been the president of the German athletics association during Arne's athletics career.

Arne succeeded in persuading the IAAF to ban anabolic steroids so that drug testing could be carried out in Rome. Two years later, the IOC also banned steroids.

Drug-testing methods remained primitive, however. 'The first tests that were carried out in Rome weren't scientifically or legally validated. The tests were primarily carried out in order to gain experience. By the 1976 Montreal Olympics, the methods we were using were so good that eight competitors were disqualified after failing drugs tests. One of them was a track and field athlete and the other seven were weightlifters. It was tempting to draw the conclusion that it was mainly weightlifters who were doping.

'But a year later, three Finnish track and field athletes tested positive, two throwers and one high jumper. That dispelled the myth completely.'

To begin with, all the tests were sent to the same laboratory in London. The ambition was to have approved testing laboratories in all countries where major competitions were being held. By the late 1970s, Arne initiated the establishment of a laboratory in Sweden. He approached the Karolinska Institutet where he, at that time, was both professor and vice-pro-chancellor.

'The Karolinska Institutet was of course a guarantee of my scientific competence and contributed to the fact that people listened to me on these issues. No other figure in the world of athletics management was of the same academic calibre. I contacted Jan Sjövall, who was then the professor of Medical Biochemistry at KI. He was a leading scientist in mass spectrometry, an analytical technique that was used to trace hormones of different composition. We were already world leaders in this technique which was a further development of mass fragmentography.

'This in turn had been developed at KI by, among others, one of my former teachers, Bo Holmstedt. Sjövall advised me to contact one of his former research students, Ingemar Björkhem, who was based at KI's new university hospital in Huddinge, south of Stockholm. This was a hospital that I had contributed to establishing in my role as vice-dean at KI and head of the Medical Programme.

'Björkhem jumped at my suggestion because it wasn't just about tracing hormones but all kinds of stimulants. Huddinge had just been assigned to carry out drug testing within the field of clinical pharmacology by Stockholm county council's health authority. This suited us perfectly.'

In 1976 Arne was elected onto the board of the IAAF. At his own suggestion, he was given the task of building up the federation's work to combat doping. The work that he had previously undertaken on a national level could now be extended internationally. Through Arne's work, the IAAF would soon become the leading international sports federation in the fight against doping, and has remained so.

'My position on the board of the IAAF gave me access both to the national athletics federations around the world and to the drug-testing laboratories in London and in Cologne, which were the best in the world in this field, headed by Arnold Beckett and Manfred Donike. I recruited both of them to the IAAF's Medical Committee.

'They were already members of the IOC's Medical Committee but the IOC's work against performance-enhancing substances could, in practice, only be carried out every fourth year in conjunction with the Olympics. They were therefore more than willing to participate in the IAAF's all-year-round work against doping. Both of them were world authorities: Beckett specialised in ephedrine research and Donike within the analysis of performance-enhancing substances. I was the only scientist with a platform within international athletics management. You could say that it was the three of us who really initiated the international fight against doping.

'Within the IAAF we developed a procedure of accreditation for drug-testing laboratories. The difference from the analysis performed in a normal hospital lab is that the result from a sports drug-test analysis is the sole evidence and has to be legally valid. This placed specific demands on the laboratory. The model for these labs was the Olympic laboratories which the IOC set up for the Olympic Games.'

Beckett and Donike were hired as experts for this process.

'They rarely agreed, except on one point; and that was that all accredited laboratories were to undergo a yearly quality control. This might sound obvious now, but it wasn't then. Many directors of the drug-testing laboratories that became accredited viewed us as some kind of police whose job was to question their competence.'

Through an agreement between Arne and the chairman of the IOC's medical committee, the Belgian Prince Alexandre de Mérode, the responsibility for accreditation of laboratories was taken over by the IOC in 1983. The aim of this was to emphasise that it was not just athletics that was subject to drug tests but every international sports federation. Today the accreditation is run by WADA, the World Anti-Doping Agency.

Steroids: The First Battle

THE SIMPLE QUESTIONNAIRE on doping that Arne had sent to the leading athletes in Sweden in 1972 had, within a decade, proved to be a snowball that turned into an avalanche. It had become obvious that steroids and other performance-enhancing substances should be prohibited within sport. A drug-testing programme was in the process of being introduced at the international level, a network of accredited drug-testing laboratories was expanding, and the results that they were able to demonstrate could hold up scientifically and in a court of law. A debate, both for and against doping, was in full swing. The majority of Swedish athletes now accepted Arne Ljungqvist's argument. The opposition that had shown itself in Halle had evaporated.

'But simultaneously we were beginning to understand in Sweden that there was a use of steroids in the country that was not only linked to sport. Maybe the use of steroids was bigger at this point outside the world of sport.'

By the end of the 1970s, the public started to have a new perception of the human body and Swedes were among the first to want to 'get in shape', following fitness shows on television. Working-out in front of fitness dance programmes and dressed in colourful sports clothes entered the nation's living rooms. The public developed a fixation about their bodies that had previously only been nurtured by bodybuilders.

Health food stores now marketed supplements not only to bodybuilders but also to people simply keen to improve their fitness. The boundary between supplements and drugs was as unclear outside the world of sport as it was within it. The sale and the use of steroids was an everyday occurrence at local gyms. And the gym was outside the jurisdiction and mandate of the Swedish Sports Confederation.

'So that became the next stage here in Sweden. We discovered that a large part of the black market trade in steroids was happening in gyms, with drugs that had been smuggled into the country and sold illegally, so we began a co-operation with the Swedish customs, the police and the National Board of Health and Welfare.

'In 1991, after a long investigation, Sweden became one of the first countries in the world to introduce a specific law criminalising the trade and possession of doping substances. It came into force on July 1, 1992 and in 1999 the law was extended to incorporate the use of these banned substances.'

Chapter 5

The Sports Official

FOR THE NEXT thirty years or so, from his office at the Karolinska Institutet, Arne ran his campaign against doping. He had the full support of his bosses and was able to combine his work against doping with the research he undertook on kidneys and renal circulation, the heart, blood vessels and cancer.

Gradually, more people began to realise that doping needed to be dealt with, and Arne Ljungqvist, his medical qualifications and experience, were much in demand. He soon found himself on the board of the Swedish Sports Confederation, and this was followed a year later by his election to the governing council of the IAAF. But as well as the new opportunities these positions afforded Arne, they also presented new dangers.

Because of his profession, Arne was already used to working in an international environment. This was to stand him in good stead as he began to move among the higher echelons of international sport. He had already learned a number of lessons during his time with the Swedish athletics association. It was a relatively small board, and the president since 1965 was a leading industrialist, Matts Carlgren.

'Up until 1970 there was no European Athletics Association, just a committee responsible for European issues within the IAAF.

'Sweden had a representative on this committee and in the IAAF – Jacob Lindahl, a former athlete, who was a decent sort of chap and very highly respected. He had previously been a member of the board of the Swedish athletics association but after stepping down had only his international duties.'

Problems arose, however, with the decision in 1970 to form the European Athletics Association, or EAA. Given his experience of issues within international athletics, and also because of his background as a former athlete, Jacob Lindahl seemed to be the natural choice for Sweden's representative on the new EAA council. Matts Carlgren had other ideas, however, and he demanded that he should be nominated for the post.

'In many ways I liked Matts, but this concerned me. I knew very well that Matts wasn't particularly known in the world of athletics.

'He was a good tennis player and had done quite a bit of long jumping as well as sprinting; but only at national level. Among the heads of international athletics, he was barely known.

'Nonetheless, Sweden still nominated him, but he failed to be elected. This meant that Sweden missed out on a place on the council of the EAA.'

The episode gave Arne a very useful insight into how appointments were made in international athletics.

His next important lesson came at the 1972 Olympics in Munich. 'The IAAF held a congress in Munich that year, and new people were to be elected on to its council. The Norwegians nominated the president of the Norwegian federation and the Danes nominated their general secretary. The Swedes, however, having learned their lesson, did not nominate Matts Carlgren this time.

'Instead Jacob Lindahl was Sweden's candidate, as he was already on the council. The Finns also supported Lindahl, and because we realised that the Nordic countries would never get three members on to the IAAF council at the same time, Lindahl was the obvious Nordic choice.

'But the Norwegian and Dane had their own ambitions, and because their federations supported them, the Nordic votes were split. Jacob was eventually the one voted in, but as the last representative and with the least votes. This is what can happen behind the scenes in the higher echelons of international athletics organisations.'

When he took over as president of the Swedish athletics association, Arne took it upon himself to strengthen the position of the Nordic nations internationally, to avoid repeating the split vote they had in Munich.

'Both the Lindahl incident and the Carlgren *faux pas* had shown the importance of strengthening the management of Nordic athletics and of getting the Nordic countries to work together and not oppose each other. This strategy should be seen in the light of the political situation in the world at the time, with clear bloc formations.'

Arne decided to forge closer ties with Finland, which was the most successful Nordic country in athletics. The idea was that a Finnish candidate would be introduced when Jacob Lindahl stepped down, which he intended to do in 1976.

'So I went and visited Jukka Uunila, who was then the most powerful figure in Finnish athletics and president of the Finnish athletics association. Outside of athletics he worked as the director of Finland's state betting company. His shortcoming internationally was that he could speak only Finnish. But I took the opportunity of his fiftieth birthday to go over and meet him.

'It is important to remember that Sweden and Finland have not always had the best relationship in sport, but I took the liberty of going as a newly appointed president. As it turned out, I was the only foreigner at Jukka's birthday party. This had an impact, as I later discovered. Jukka was delighted and this led us to begin discussing who we would nominate to the council of the IAAF at the 1976 congress in Montreal.'

Arne and Jukka agreed to organise a meeting of the Nordic associations on the island of Åland. There, they agreed a set of guidelines for what was to become a huge success for the Nordic countries, first at the IAAF congress staged in conjunction with the Olympic Games, and at subsequent congresses. For Arne, it resulted in him being elected to the IAAF council.

'Nordic representatives went on to chair four of the IAAF's six committees. A Dane became chair of the race walking committee, another Dane head of the technical committee, a Norwegian was head of the masters' committee and I headed the medical committee. This was an amazing success.'

When an election was held for the EAA council, a Finn was elected. All this was a result of what the Nordic countries had agreed on at the meeting in Åland in 1975. 'It was thanks to that event that we held a number of prominent positions within the running of international athletics.

'This was such a success that Primo Nebiolo, who was a master of intrigues and who would go on to be IAAF president in 1981, came to me one day and asked: "How the hell have you done this? You are completely over-represented."'

Back at home in Sweden, Arne was also busy sorting things out and recruiting the people he wanted for the Swedish athletics association. When he was elected, the general secretary left with a pension. Ulf Ekelund was recruited as the replacement, a post he would hold until 1993, when he moved on to run the local organising committee for the 1995 IAAF world championships in Gothenburg.

However, not everyone immediately supported Ulf. 'My view was that if anyone could, Ulf would help give the media a fresh view of Swedish athletics. Our relationship with the media had left a lot to be desired for many years, and now we were heading into an era when it was becoming all the more important to be visible to the public. I wanted to put the Swedish athletics association on the map, at home and internationally.

'But then we had a very poor national team. We were always being beaten by the Finns, who were better across all the events, and we had very few international stars. We also had problems with recruitment.

'The best athletes wanted to go in to football or ice hockey, while no one was interested in athletics, where our competitors from East Germany, the Soviet Union and the United States were, with the help of performance-enhancing substances, producing performances to a level that was unreachable. I think that this was a big part of it. It would later be revealed that many of the stars gained their star status by using steroids, with a few exceptions.'

But among the Swedish stars there was one who shone more brightly than most. She was known as 'the pin-up girl of Swedish athletics', a beautiful and unusually gifted sprinter, Linda Haglund. Haglund was the only one who challenged the Eastern bloc's dominance.

Linda Haglund's popularity in the late 1970s can be compared to Carolina Klüft's popularity today. She would have outshone both Anja Persson and Susanna Kallur. Her career ran parallel with Arne's: she won 60-metres gold at the European Indoor Championships in 1976, 100-metres silver at the European Championships in Prague two years later, and she was fourth in the 100 metres at the 1980 Moscow Olympic Games.

The glory of her success was also reflected on the Swedish athletics association. You could be forgiven for thinking that this was the fruit of the new president's labours. As it turned out, it was because of something else entirely.

TOWARDS THE END of the 1981 track season, Linda was due to participate in the World Cup in Rome as a member of the European team. Arne had at this point handed over the presidency to Hans Holmér, but was nonetheless present in Rome as part of the delegation at the IAAF's congress.

While there, Ulf Ekelund called Arne to a meeting. It was then that he dropped a bombshell. Linda Haglund had tested positive for steroids. The tests had been conducted at the Swedish championships some weeks earlier.

'I knew what it was about as I had been given confidential information by Ulf that Linda had been given steroids by mistake by her trainer, Pertti Helin. And now the analytical result had confirmed that she was positive.

'Ekelund and I agreed that Linda should be withdrawn from the European team under the pretext that she was injured. It was a half-truth, but we decided to go with this in order not to damage the team during a competition.'

But Linda Haglund's positive drug test was also hushed up after the competition. This was in spite of the fact that Arne urged Holmér to tell the media the truth. 'He categorically refused and was of the opinion that we should keep quiet about it for as long as possible. I had to trust him: he was, after all, a lawyer and came directly from his post as head of the Swedish security police.

'I thought he knew what he was talking about. It was he, after all, who would have to deal with it as president of the Swedish association. Or so I thought.'

Arne wondered what he ought to say if someone asked him a direct question. 'Then we tell it like it is,' he was told.

'I thought that it would have been better to be straight about what had happened from the beginning, instead of hushing it up. But it was Hans Holmér who had the final say. And when the truth finally leaked out, it was massive front page news like never before.'

What followed was pure drama.

Massive portions of the media and general public took Linda's side. Linda was seen to have been tricked into taking steroids by Pertti Helin, her Finnish coach. She was supposed to have been given the tablets to treat a bad back or something similar, and he was supposed to have told her that it was vitamins, which was supposed to help. The investigation that the Swedish Sports Confederation implemented seemed to confirm this version of events.

The steroids had been kept in a bottle labelled as some medication which did not contain any banned substance.

Helin could not give any satisfactory explanation as to why on earth he had steroids in such a bottle.

'So Linda was cleared by the board of the Swedish athletics association and was seen as having been tricked by her trainer. But Pertti Helin was also cleared by the Finns.

'So we had our first case where an athlete had tested positive but no one was found guilty.'

The situation was unacceptable as far as the IAAF was concerned and when the Nordic athletics associations held their annual meeting, which took place in Oslo in 1981, Arne raised the issue and encouraged the Finnish and Swedish associations to reconsider their decision. They refused.

So Arne then began to explore the possibility of the IAAF re-examining the findings of the national associations, but that, too, proved impossible. 'The case concerned a national competition, which meant that the IAAF had no say in the matter according to the IAAF general secretary John Holt.

'He interpreted the rules in such a way that it was up to the respective national associations to convict or, in this case, clear them, as they saw fit. The only thing the IAAF could do, according to the general secretary, was to take action against the Swedish and Finnish associations directly as members of the IAAF.'

Despite the inadequate regulations and general secretary's ruling, the IAAF council decided to ban Linda Haglund for eighteen months and it called on the Finnish federation to ban Pertti Helin. This was a ruling Arne had helped push through, although he abstained from taking part in the decision because he was too involved in the case.

'You might wonder why we didn't go harder after Pertti Helin, but we really didn't have any jurisdiction in the matter. Back then there was no possibility for the IAAF to ban a coach; that rule was only introduced at the end of the 1980s.'

Linda appealed against the IAAF ban and her case was taken up the following year at the IAAF council meeting in Kingston, Jamaica. Both Linda Haglund and Hans Holmér attended to put forward Haglund's case, but it didn't help: the ban remained in place. Linda Haglund's career was over.

She made an attempt at a comeback after the ban was lifted, but it didn't work. And the Finns finally fired Helin.

THE HAGLUND SAGA had put Arne back in the glare of the media spotlight. 'I managed to put the entire Swedish athletics association, of which I had been head of for almost ten years, against me.

'The Swedish daily newspaper *Dagens Nyheter* published an open letter to me, which was signed by Linda Haglund but most probably written by Holmér. I was slammed for not having hurried to her defence in "this dreadful legal assault", as she put it. But I was convinced that if we had let Linda and her Finnish coach go unpunished, the anti-doping campaign would have been dead in the water.

'It would have meant that whoever tested positive for doping would be able to put the blame on someone in their camp who could take the blame instead and claim that they had tricked the athlete into taking steroids or other performance-enhancing substances. It just wasn't on.

'Sure, I was prepared that something like this would happen. As soon as I started working against doping I realised that a major Swedish star would sooner or later get caught. I understood that it would be difficult and that there would be a lot of flak.'

There was indeed. Holmér didn't give up and speculation about Linda's own culpability wouldn't die down. Finally, a journalist at Swedish tabloid *Expressen*, Lennart Eriksson, patched together a very unlikely conspiracy theory which was published in November 1983.

'According to Eriksson I was meant to have knowingly tried to sweep the whole incident under the carpet, only to have then changed my mind and let down my own colleagues when the story broke.

'I hit the roof. I called up Bo Strömstedt, the chief editor at *Expressen*, but he had already formed his opinion, like many others, and reckoned I was up to no good.

'The worst thing about it was being called a liar when I tried to respond to the accusations that were being levelled against me. In the end I contacted one of Sweden's top lawyers who specialised in the freedom of the press and libel cases. When we met I asked him if I was being libelled, and he told me I was. When I asked him if I would win a defamation case if I went to court he told me I would.

'But when I asked him if we should do it, he told me most definitely not.'

The lawyer sketched out a scenario where Arne would find himself even more under the media spotlight without any chance of defending himself.

'If we do nothing, the whole story will quickly be forgotten and be totally uninteresting. *Expressen* has everything to gain by keeping the story alive, selling newspapers about the court case.'

So Arne didn't take the matter to court. And there still doesn't exist any Swedish disciplinary action against Linda Haglund. But the Haglund case saw a significant change in international sport's anti-doping rules, the principle of 'strict liability', which remains to this day enshrined in the World Anti-Doping Agency's code.

Under the 'strict liability' principle, it is the sole responsibility of an athlete to ensure that they do not take banned substances. No competitor can claim that another person has tricked them into taking a banned substance or that they consumed the banned substance by accident, for example, through contaminated food or food supplements. Thus, any athlete who tests positive for a banned substance will be disqualified and banned from competing, no matter how the substance got into their body.

The debate that raged in Sweden concerning Linda Haglund dragged the question of doping into the spotlight, which helped to contribute to more immediate changes, and as early as 1982, random, out-of-competition testing was introduced for Swedish athletes even during the closed season – nearly a decade earlier than in the rest of the world.

'I took the whole thing with Linda Haglund very hard. This was maybe because people that I thought were my friends acted so strangely. I later renewed my contact with Hans Holmér, although we never spoke of the Haglund case. I got a lot of good support from Hans during my years as president of the Swedish Sports Confederation between 1989 and 2001.

'Even Ulf Ekelund remained one of my good friends. As for Linda, I must tell you what happened at the first Swedish Sports Gala at the Stockholm Globe Arena in 2000.

'We hadn't seen each other since that meeting in Jamaica nineteen years earlier when she and Holmér had attempted to prove her innocence. So I am sitting there, watching the stage when someone taps me on the shoulder. I turn around and Linda is standing there. She greets me and then gives me a hug.

'I was so touched by her gesture. It says a lot about Linda Haglund as a person. I have seen her a few times since then.'

Chapter 6

The King, the Prince and I

ARNE LJUNGQVIST WAS forty years old when elected to the board of the Swedish athletics association in 1971. It was a timely appointment, because no one at the athletics association had his kind of medical qualifications and experience. The need for someone to tackle the issue of drugs in sport was increasingly evident, and so it was not long before Arne found himself also elected to the board of the Swedish Sports Confederation.

The Swedish Sports Confederation is an umbrella-organisation which covers all the national sports federations, both Olympic and non-Olympic. The Swedish Olympic Committee (SOK) is solely responsible for planning and managing Sweden's participation in the Olympic Games. The government-funded Swedish Sports Confederation, on the other hand, is responsible for formulating the policy for Swedish sport.

During the mid-1970s, the confederation itself and its ruling board were chaired by different people. The president of the confederation was Prince Bertil, his vice-president was the speaker from the Swedish parliament, Ingemund Bengstsson.

Meanwhile, the chairman of the confederation's board was Kalle Frithiofson, once a social democrat politician who from 1975 was the governor of a county in western Sweden. It was when Arne replaced Frithiofson in 1989 that he was unexpectedly summoned to meet Prince Bertil at Stockholm's Royal Palace. The prince didn't beat about the bush.

'Now,' he said. 'Ingemund and I have agreed that it's time to modernise the leadership of Swedish sport. The chairman of the board of the Swedish Sports Confederation is now to be the president of the confederation itself. So, I'm resigning and you're taking over.'

The news came as a complete surprise for Arne. 'I thought it strange to replace the prince, so I objected, saying I didn't think it was a very good suggestion. But the prince insisted: "Ingemund and I have decided that you should take the position."

'So I accepted with due grace. Suddenly I was not only chairman of the board of the Sports Confederation but also president of the Swedish Sports Confederation, the first non-royal person in Swedish history to have that position.'

PRINCE BERTIL WAS nicknamed 'the Prince of Sport', and sometimes 'the Turbo Prince'. He had a profound interest in sport. It was probably Bo Ekelund, the ex-chairman of the Swedish athletics association and industrialist, who had told him about Arne.

Ekelund had held high positions in a number of Swedish and international sporting associations. Like Arne he, too, had also previously been a high jumper. 'He clearly kept an eye on me; it was evident quite early on. As he was a close friend of Prince Bertil, I presume it was he who put a good word in for me.

'They both supported me a lot during my career. The prince never told me directly why he selected me, but in a number of different ways he led me to believe this was the case.'

Arne became very close to the prince. 'He was an incredibly nice person. Very amenable. It's easy to understand why he was well-liked by the people. When you sat talking to him you were constantly on the verge of addressing him using "Du" – the informal way Swedish friends and family address each other. He was like a friend you talked to, and you sensed he was quite at home among sportsmen and sportswomen.

'Prince Bertil was a kind of substitute father for his nephew, Carl Gustaf, now King of Sweden, whose father, Bertil's older brother Prince Gustaf Adolf, was killed in an air crash when Carl Gustaf was still a baby. I know for a fact that the Swedish King and Queen were deeply grateful for what he did for them.'

Towards the end of Prince Bertil's life, Arne was often by his side, regularly visiting Villa Solbacken, the home of Prince Bertil and his wife Princess Lilian. The prince walked with a walking frame after suffering a fall from a stepladder. After the accident, he was never quite the same and withdrew from public life.

'He didn't want to appear incapacitated in public. Every time I visited him at home, a couple of times each year, he always expected fresh reports from the world of sport. I really felt like a close friend of the prince.'

Arne's 'promotion' wasn't just an honour for him but very significant in terms of his international sporting network.

Arne was digging in the garden of his home in Enebyberg, just north of Stockholm one day in 1976 when

Ulla, his wife, put her head out the window and called out that the marshal of the realm was on the phone.

'At first, I just thought it was one of my brothers mucking about. So I plodded in slowly with my wellington boots on and lifted up the receiver, my hands covered in mud.

'But it really was the marshal of the realm. He had a question. Would I agree to be one of the King's chamberlains? I felt that I was completely inappropriately dressed for a conversation of this kind.'

At that time there was about twelve King's chamberlains in Sweden. They are appointed by the King and are responsible for assisting him at major receptions and dinners, like 'assistant hosts'. They help welcome the guests and ensure that they are enjoying themselves. The King's chamberlains also participate when new ambassadors of foreign countries hand in their credentials at their first visit to the King, and when heads of state make official visits to Sweden. To be selected is a civil honour, comparable with the military honour of *aide de camp*, which is awarded by the armed forces.

Traditionally, the King's chamberlains have been selected from the royal family's friends and were often from the nobility. 'I understood that the new King wanted to modernise and widen the scope of the chamberlains by bringing in people, as in my case, from the worlds of sport and science. I am completely convinced that Prince Bertil was behind this move, too.'

The King's chamberlains wear a special uniform: a dress coat with gold buttons and gold braid. 'I bought a used one from chamberlain Crispin Löwenhielm when he was "discharged". It had to be adjusted to fit me. The tailor told me that a new chamberlain uniform costs more than 40,000 Swedish kronor, more than 5,000 US dollars at 2010 exchange rates. The uniform was also accompanied by a hat which costs several thousand kronor more, so it's fair to say that it's very expensive to play the role of a King's chamberlain! But I got to sell the whole caboodle back to the court when I left in 2001, when I turned seventy, though I keep the title and some privileges.

'I always wore the uniform when ambassadors from around the world came to hand in their credentials and on other state occasions. The King also wanted us to wear the uniform when he celebrated his fiftieth birthday. Otherwise, you wear a jacket embossed with the King's name and gold buttons instead. This was what I usually wore at dinners and mingling at the royal palace. You wear a dark suit for informal gatherings.'

After several years as one of the King's chamberlains, in 1986 Arne was promoted to be a lord-in-waiting at the court. This meant that Arne was required to stay at the palace overnight during state visits and be involved in hosting the visiting heads of state. There are only three or four lords-in-waiting. Arne met many world leaders during his years of service, when meeting royalty and celebrities became a part of his everyday life. But the appointment was very fruitful for making international contacts.

'I remember in particular the Japanese Emperor and his wife, who I got quite close to. Crown Prince Akihito and Crown Princess Michiko made an official visit to Stockholm in 1985, several years before he was crowned emperor, and then came back on a state visit in 2000. My eldest son had lived and worked in Japan for several years; he spoke Japanese and also had a PhD from the University of Tokyo. I knew from what he said how revered the emperor was and how the emperor had previously been so hidden from the public.

'The Emperor Akihito and his wife had broken that tradition and were seen increasingly in public. By ceasing to be so aloof, they made themselves much more well-liked; I could understand it, too, because of their friendly and inviting manner. Normally, a state visit lasts for three days, but the Emperor and his wife arrived a day early and invited me to tea. They were staying at Haga Slott, a palace just outside Stockholm. They were going to stay at the Royal Palace when the official state visit commenced.

'Now they wanted to get to know me and two others: a lady-in-waiting and an *aide de camp*. When I mentioned my son's interest in Japan, they were very enthusiastic.

'Queen Beatrix of the Netherlands was also a surprisingly pleasant acquaintance. She was a spontaneous and delightful lady who, after her farewell banquet, once the official business was over, invited me to a party at the palace. It ended with us sitting into the early hours of the morning, drinking champagne and talking. It was a very pleasant occasion where I had the opportunity to tell her about Sweden, sport and myself.'

After his many years of working in the Swedish court, Arne is well-known to his country's royal family. 'It's formal when things are meant to be formal like during state visits, banquets or other official engagements. But if we meet in the stadium stands or, as we did at the Athens Olympic Games in 2004, we meet up in the hotel bar to celebrate the Swedish gold medals, then it is like talking to anyone. It's not like I address the King using the familiar "du", but apart from that it's just like talking to a regular person.

'And that's just how the royal couple want it, as far as I understand. The same goes for their children. It's very easy to talk to them. Very pleasant.'

It is well-known in Sweden how much King Carl Gustaf and Queen Silvia become involved in sporting events when they are sitting in the stands. 'I remember when Stefan Holm won the high jump at the Athens Olympics. I thought the King was going to explode. I understood then that the royal family's interest in sport isn't made up: it's spontaneous and very genuine.

'Besides, both the King and Queen are very knowledgeable when it comes to sport. It's fun to represent Swedish sport in their presence.'

THROUGH HIS INVOLVEMENT in international athletics, Arne has also met many other celebrities, including Prince Albert of Monaco. 'I know Prince Albert very well, and have met his whole family. He is an IOC member.

'He was an Olympian himself, having competed in the bobsleigh. I think that is why he feels so relaxed when he is in our company and can escape from the glare of the media. He is also the honorary chairman of the board of the IAAF Foundation of which I am vice-chairman. It is a small board with just eleven members. It hands out about million dollars each year to different sporting projects.

'The board was created after the Seoul Olympics in South Korea in 1988. Prince Albert always attends our meetings and he is a dreadfully nice person and knowledgeable sportsman.'

Another figure Arne has met is Britain's Prince Philip. 'The Swedish Sports Confederation had a meeting with their British counterparts – then called the Sports Council – at the end of the 1970s. The meeting was to take place at Buckingham Palace.

'Our delegation was headed by Prince Bertil and we were to be met by a member of royalty of similar rank. As it turned out, it was Prince Philip, who was then the president of the International Equestrian Federation, before his daughter Princess Anne took over.

'Prince Philip led our meetings with enormous stringency and utter professionalism. I was pleasantly surprised because I had only had his media image to go on before then. This all happened very early on in my career as a sports official at this level and naturally, I was impressed. Over the years I got used to working in this kind of environment and the people there, but back then it was really something special to sit at Buckingham Palace and be offered lunch by the British royal family.'

A third major figure Arne encountered was Henri, Grand Duke of Luxembourg, who over the years became a good friend. Just because Prince Bertil once turned down the opportunity to be a member of the IOC on the basis that he believed the committee shouldn't just be known for its royal members that did not stop other royals from joining the IOC.

Grand Duke Henri is one of them. He 'inherited' the post from his father, Grand Duke Jean. His mother, the Grand Duchess Josephine Charlotte of Belgium, was half Swedish, the daughter of Leopold III of Belgium and Astrid of Sweden.

'Because he is an IOC member, we meet quite regularly, and he's always the first to come over to me. I use a protocol at the IOC that says that royalty approach me first, and not the other way around. So Henri always comes over and says hello. Again, my eldest son is a bit of connection because after his years in Japan, he moved to Luxembourg where he lived with his family for ten years. I have a standing invitation from the Grand Duke to get in touch when I am there and go out and have lunch together with our families.'

Yet of all the people Arne has met, it is his time with Nelson Mandela that he values most of all. In 1996, the IAAF organised its world cross-country championships in South Africa for the first time, in Cape Town. 'Mandela is one person I would never have got to meet if it hadn't been for sport. He was, as everyone says, a very friendly person. His whole being oozes friendliness. A few of us from the IAAF council got to meet him. He was very particular in asking who we were and who I knew in Sweden. He asked me to send his best wishes to the Swedish prime minister Ingvar Carlsson. I know he liked Ingvar Carlsson and the feeling was mutual.

'At lunch one day I got to sit next to one of Mandela's colleagues. I think he was the minister for youth and sport, I can't quite remember his name. I knew that he had been a prisoner along with Mandela at Robben Island for twenty-seven years. So I asked him how they could be so forgiving towards their captors. He answered that it was a strategy they decided on very early on at Robben Island. It was the only way South Africa would avoid a civil war. That they went on to succeed was thanks to the way they decided to pursue reconciliation and forgiveness.

'Mandela gave me a photograph of himself in his prison cell. I have it on a wall at home. I was also given a copy of his book, signed, where he outlines how people can peacefully co-exist in South Africa.'

THE NETWORK OF well-placed, international contacts that Arne built thanks to his positions at the Swedish court and in international sport also put him in contact with a few less salubrious people.

Ferdinand Marcos, the infamous former president of the Philippines, was among those. 'The IAAF had its council meeting in Manila and we were invited on board a private jet which flew us to the then president's summer residence up in the mountains in the north of the Philippines. The president and his wife were notorious around the world. I spent a day with them. The president looked really ill. Imelda Marcos, on the other hand, gave a quite different impression. It was very clear who wore the trousers in that relationship.

'Another time I met the then Prime Minister of Italy, Bettino Craxi. He was later charged with corruption and fled to Tunisia. He awarded the members of the council of the IAAF a rather unusual Italian order of merit. I usually wear it when I attend banquets and receptions at the royal palace. When people ask me what kind of order it is, I tell them that I was awarded it by Bettino Craxi. That always makes them step back in surprise.

'I met the Romanian dictator Nicolae Ceauscescu as well. This was in 1980, during my time as the King's chamberlain. I wasn't staying at the royal palace during his state visit, I just met him during the day. At the start of the 1970s a Romanian researcher on a scholarship worked at my lab at Karolinska for a year. They rarely let anyone out of the country, let alone researchers, but I wanted this doctoral student back to finish off certain projects. I had worked quite hard to get him out through the official channels, but it was proving hopeless.

'So during Ceauscescu's state visit, I took up the matter with his personal physician, who was accompanying him. Nothing came of it though. The Romanian regime was unyielding. Looking back at that state visit, it is obvious it wasn't among the most pleasant. But the royal court had no say in deciding who was socially acceptable and who wasn't. Their hands were tied by the Swedish Foreign Ministry, and they followed international protocol which regulates the choice of state visits.'

The example of Arne's meeting with Nicolae Ceauscescu doesn't just illustrate the more disagreeable duties that the King's chamberlain had to cope with. It also exemplifies a problem which Arne was confronted with again and again during his years at the IOC and IAAF: boycotts.

There were repeated calls for the boycott of some country or other from upset people. And time and again, some country or other decided to boycott a particular event or championship.

'But why boycott one dictator but not another? Where do you draw the line? And at what point do we risk isolating ourselves? Ceauscescu was a dictator. So is Castro in Cuba, Marcos in the Philippines, and that's not even mentioning the leadership in the Soviet Union. It is easy to sit here in judgement years later. Sure, it is perhaps questionable that Ceauscescu was awarded the Swedish Order of the Seraphim as a visiting head of state. But such was the protocol.

'The events of Los Angeles in 1984 should not be forgotten, when the entire Eastern bloc boycotted the Olympics, except Romania, which wanted to draw attention to its independence. Then, they were applauded by the majority of the sporting world.

'I had a very clear picture of what the situation was like in Romania. My doctoral student had recounted things to me about the totalitarian regime there that only became widely understood after Ceauscescu was deposed in 1989.

'I do not think boycotts work. I would rather stress the colossal significance of sport as a peaceful bridge between nations. Sport is so important to each country in spite of its political structure. There are lots of examples of how sport opens doors.'

SPORT AND SCIENCE HAVE GONE hand in hand during Arne's entire career. His senior position at the world-renowned Karolinska Institutet has more than once been of benefit to his work within sport. There are, however, also examples of how his involvement in sport has opened doors for him as a scientist – doors that might otherwise have been hermetically sealed.

In 1978, Arne was the chairman of the Medical Studies Commission at Karolinska and so responsible for the medical curriculum. When attending a medical conference, he told an American colleague about his work. The colleague recommended that Arne go to China. 'They're at the cutting edge,' he told Arne. The American had just been there on a group visit for American university lecturers and returned with many new discoveries.

'There were so many dreadful restrictions if you wanted to travel to China then. This was right after the so-called "Gang of Four". You only got a visa to visit China if you were travelling in a group, like a delegation.' But it wasn't possible for Arne to arrange a whole delegation.

Instead, Arne walked over to the Chinese consulate in Stockholm. In his briefcase he had all the recommendations and references he had managed to scrape together, one of them rubber stamped by Jan-Erik Wikström, the Education Minister. His briefcase also contained documents from the University's Chancellery and from the Karolinska Institutet.

'Then I thought "What the hell," and I threw in all my documents related to my career as an athlete and sports leader. At the consulate, a senior civil servant sat there going through my papers and rubber-stamped documents. It wasn't working. Not until he saw the things from my involvement in sport. "This looks very interesting," he said, and promised to get back to me.

'Three weeks later, my application for an entry visa to go to study the Chinese medical training programme had been transformed to an official, personal invitation from the Chinese state, hosted by the All China Sports Federation. They offered me the opportunity to study anything related to sport and medical science and education. Clearly, the merits that I had gained through my involvement in sport opened the door.'

Chapter 7

Nebiolo, Samaranch and I

THE SAME YEAR of 1976 that Arne Ljungqvist was elected on to what was then the International Amateur Athletics Federation's ruling council, saw the Dutchman, Adriaan Paulen take over as President from Lord Burghley.

From the long list of candidates from around the world nominated for a place on the board, Arne was elected with the most votes. The candidate who was elected at the same time with the lowest number of votes was an Italian. 'Isn't Italy in Europe anymore?' he cried indignantly when it was clear he had scraped in by just one vote and that many European countries had not voted for him.

'If that vote hadn't gone to Primo Nebiolo, the world of sport would look very different today, I can promise you.

'How on earth he got on to the board, I don't know. Nebiolo was disliked by many, and he knew it.'

Then, as now, the presidency of the athletics world governing body is among the most influential in international sport. With athletics being the centrepiece of the summer Olympic Games, the IAAF president is widely regarded as the third-most important global sporting official after the president of the IOC itself and the head of FIFA, football's world body.

Once elected on to the IAAF council, Primo Nebiolo set about digging his way into the organisation. There were no rules that he could not work his way around. Very early on it became apparent to the other council members that Nebiolo was running some kind of underground operation with the sole purpose of getting himself elected president of the IAAF.

'Long before he was elected, there were rumours he had ambitions to lead the IAAF. Now we got to see how he worked to fulfil his ambitions, with no expense spared. As early as 1979, proposals started to reach me, particularly from European representatives. They wanted me to be ready to stand against Nebiolo as a candidate for president when that day came. They also promised to work to convince the rest of the world to ensure that I would win the vote.'

Adriaan Paulen had intended to be re-elected at the 1980 Congress and as long as Paulen was willing to stand, Arne resisted all appeals for him to oppose Nebiolo in an election.

What Paulen didn't see, though, was that he was on course to lose the election before it had ever taken place.

The IAAF Congress was to be held in conjunction with the 1980 Olympic Games in Moscow, but as many countries boycotted those Olympics, the Congress was postponed. This decision played into Nebiolo's hands. Despite being only a member of the council, Nebiolo took it upon himself to set up an extra Congress, to be staged on his home turf in Rome the following year.

'There was an ingenious game of intrigue behind the extra Congress, and poor Paulen just didn't get it. He didn't understand what was brewing until it was too late.' When Paulen finally realised that Nebiolo had seized the initiative, it was too late for Arne to launch his candidacy.

'There was a lot of pressure from different quarters in Europe that I should stand. It was too late, though, for me to begin any kind of campaign. Besides, I hadn't even turned fifty and I had my career as a researcher to think about. I had become pro-vice-chancellor of the Karolinska Institutet and had a lot of other irons in the fire. Being head of the IAAF is a full-time job, so that would have meant chucking everything else aside. So I said no.

'But Nebiolo didn't know this, and I am sure that even until the day he died, he never found out either. Never.

'Back in 1981, as the date of the Congress approached, he sent for me, wanting to meet on neutral ground at the Hôtel d'Angleterre in Copenhagen. There, Nebiolo sat down and began to explain that as he saw it, it wasn't good for him or for me if I stood against him. It was really amusing to sit and listen to him because he didn't have a clue that I had already decided not to stand.

'In return, he offered me the post of vice-president, but only if I promised not to stand for election. I laughed inwardly because the vice-president wasn't decided by the president but by the council. But after Nebiolo was elected, he immediately started being a dictator. And after I had been re-elected to the council, I was made vice-president, just as he'd promised.

'I am often asked if I regret my decision not to stand for president, but I always knew that I wasn't ready to dedicate my life to sport full-time. But it was a learning position and gave me a hold over Primo Nebiolo. He believed that I had done him a massive favour. And, of course, I was happy to let him keep on believing it.'

THE MODERN OLYMPIC GAMES, first staged in 1896 under the inspiration of Baron de Coubertin, had been effectively the official world championships for athletics. But by the mid-1970s and in to the early 1980s, there was a growing desire within the IAAF to create an event where the world's elite athletes could compete outside of the Olympics, especially after two Games in succession, Montreal in 1976 and Moscow in 1980, had been scarred by politically inspired boycotts.

In 1975, when Lord Burghley was still IAAF president, as a first step towards a separate athletics world championships, it was agreed to create the World Cup, which took place for the first time in Düsseldorf in 1977. It was set up as a team event between the leading athletics nations and the continents. The idea was that this would be almost a 'warm up' for the world championships, and that the World Cup would be dropped once the world championships were launched.

There were many reasons why the IAAF considered initiating its own championships in addition to the Olympics. One was the commercial aspect. Athletics was the central feature of the Olympic Games and attracted millions of dollars in sponsorship. Boycotts were another important consideration, especially after almost all the African countries were absent from the 1976 Montreal Olympics and a large part of the West boycotted the 1980 Moscow Games. The risk of a 'revenge' boycott by the Eastern bloc of the 1984 Olympics to be staged in Los Angeles was very well anticipated in the years after Moscow.

The IAAF did not want a world championships where half of the nations would not participate. For example, when there was a boycott of the 1976 Olympics in protest over some countries' continuing links with apartheid

South Africa. The only African nation to compete at those Montreal Games was Senegal, something which today's president of the IAAF, Lamine Diack, a Senegalese, still takes pride in. But after the disappointing Olympic absences, the first World Cup, staged in Duesseldorf in 1977, unaffected by global politics, was regarded as such a success that the IAAF, under Adriaan Paulen, opted to keep it as a major event, staging it again in Montreal in 1979 and then Rome in 1981, while also making plans to introduce the world championships.

Athletics' first world championships were staged in Helsinki in 1983. In other words, it took place two years after Nebiolo had taken over as president. But the world championships were not launched on Nebiolo's own initiative, as he later pretended.

In fact, Nebiolo was at first afraid that an athletics world championships run by the IAAF might be seen as 'competition' for the Olympic Games, and therefore might damage his relationship with the new IOC president, Juan Antonio Samaranch.

Nebiolo was very ambitious, and he desperately wanted to be offered a place as a member of the International Olympic Committee. So he did not want anything to undermine his relationship with Samaranch.

But after 1983, when Nebiolo realised that the IAAF's world championships – the first worldwide athletics meeting for nearly two decades not to be damaged by boycotts or terrorism – were a huge success, both commercially with sponsors and television broadcasters, as well as politically with the IOC, then he did not waste any time in taking full advantage and claiming the credit.

Nebiolo was silent about the fact that the initiative for the world championships had been taken during Adriaan Paulen's presidency. 'It would never have occurred to

Nebiolo to deny any claim that he was the front figure when the world championships were created. The very idea was quite alien to him because he always supported anything that worked to his personal advantage.'

When first devised, the world championships were envisaged as being every fourth year, just like the Olympics, but in the year ahead of the Games. The second world championships were staged in Rome in 1987, the third in Tokyo in 1991.

With sponsors eagerly lining up to be involved with the IAAF's successful new event, Nebiolo saw to it that they should take place every other year. There were good sporting reasons for this, as well as commercial ones. An athlete's career is often very short, and a single missed world championships can be devastating for a competitor if they have to wait four years for their next opportunity.

The commercial success of the world championships was something Nebiolo knew about very well. He was an incredibly astute businessman, and at the IAAF, athletics were his goods. At times, he tried to play hardball to the point of foolhardiness. 'It was ahead of the world championships in Rome in 1987 that the TV companies' negotiators suddenly started approaching me to question whether Nebiolo had gone crazy. It turned out that Nebiolo was insisting on absurd conditions in conjunction with the TV rights. When I spoke to him about it he just answered: "Arne, what you have to understand is that these companies *have* to broadcast the championships."

'I realised how bloody tough and adept he was at negotiating when his demands were actually accepted. He even managed to raise the price for the contract from ten million dollars to nearly a hundred million dollars. By the time the IAAF staged its fourth world championships, in Stuttgart in 1993, he had negotiated a new Mercedes for each winner. Today, each winner at the world championships receives 60,000 US dollars and the finalists also receive prize money.

'I know that Samaranch was extremely concerned that this would spread to the Olympics. "At the Olympics," Samaranch said, "there will never be any prize money as the Olympic medal is the finest reward you can get."

'But Nebiolo's strategy to commercialise the world championships was well thought through. He knew that money is power and that money creates prestige. And he raised the prestige of athletics by showing how much money it was worth.'

PRIMO NEBIOLO WAS a tough negotiator, with an iron will and a temperament that earned him the nickname 'the dictator' even among his closest colleagues. He was also hungry for prestige, and keen to create an aura of glamour around the world of international athletics and his own person. He was also vain.

'He called himself "Doctor" Nebiolo, probably as a result of the honorary doctorates that he collected. He wanted to become an honorary doctor at every city that arranged the world championships, and he therefore had a request sent to the Finns in 1983, and to us in Sweden in connection with the world championships in Gothenburg in 1995. He pointed out that it would be appropriate for him to become an honorary doctor at the University of Helsinki and at Gothenburg University. He got a similar answer on both occasions, because Nordic countries have particular requirements for conferring an honorary doctorate on someone; of which Nebolio was probably unaware. Perhaps it's not strange then that he never really liked us up here in the north! As a consolation, in 1995 he was given the key to the city of Gothenburg instead, which the political leaders had hastily sorted out.'

The decision to establish an international athletics association was taken in conjunction with the 1912 Stockholm Olympics. Even though it was formally founded in Berlin a year later, and the Germans have consistently claimed that it was formed there and then, the IAAF celebrated its 80th anniversary in 1992 in Stockholm with a royal banquet in the Blue Hall at Stockholm City Hall.

'Nebiolo demanded that Queen Silvia should be placed next to him at his table and that the King be placed opposite him.

'To place someone other than the Queen opposite the King on such an occasion goes against royal protocol. The King and the Queen are always to be placed facing each other. I was a King's chamberlain, so the Lord Chamberlain, Kuylenstierna, turned to me and said: "Arne, you will have to fix this. This is completely impossible." I promised to do what I could, but Nebiolo persisted.

'He threatened that if he didn't get his way, he wouldn't come at all.

'The royal household became more and more anxious, and it went so far that they considered breaking protocol and giving in to his demands. But I knew that Nebiolo played against the odds when negotiating, so I firmly advised the royal family to not give in. I knew full well that Nebiolo was more than tickled by the thought of sitting next to the Queen. This was just the way he played and many of his business partners went along with it. But royal protocol was adhered to and a very satisfied Nebiolo was seated next to the Queen, but with the King at an angle from him.'

It wasn't just the seating arrangements at the table that caused problems. All the notabilities were to be housed at the Grand Hotel. Among those expected were Samaranch, who was booked in at the same time as Nebiolo and Prince Albert, who at that time was still the Crown Prince of Monaco. This was a major headache. It was self-evident that Crown Prince Albert should be given the largest suite, but the question remained what to do with Samaranch and Nebiolo.

'I think that Nebiolo could have accepted that Crown Prince Albert would be given the largest suite, but he would never have accepted Samaranch being given a larger suite than him. As it turned out, the whole thing was solved when Samaranch cancelled. But I know that the same thing or worse happened another time. It was at the world championships in Helsinki in 1983. The IOC suddenly announced that their executive board would congregate for an extra meeting in Helsinki. The reason, of course, was that the IOC was suspicious of the IAAF and they were afraid that the world championships were competing with the Olympics. They wanted to know what was going on.

'This created some logistical problems, not just in terms of finding hotel rooms and grand dinners for the sporting dignitaries. The real problem was Nebiolo and Samaranch. Who was to have the best suite? It sounds crazy and it is, but the organisers had to have the suites measured to be sure that Nebiolo was not given a smaller suite than Samaranch. How childish!

'In Helsinki another incident occurred. The IOC and Samaranch suddenly demanded that the Olympic flag should be flown on the inner athletics field during the world championships. The organisers were perplexed and the chairman of the organising committee, Carl-Olaf Homen, sought my advice. We discussed the problem and found a diplomatic solution. Carl-Olaf declared that there were only two flagpoles on the inner field (which was true) and they were not allowed more (which was not true at all).

'One of the flagpoles had to fly the Finnish flag and, of course, the other had to fly the IAAF flag. So the Olympic flag was placed on the roof of the podium where it flew alongside all the national flags, no doubt much to Samaranch's irritation.'

NEBIOLO'S VANITY OFTEN had its comic side. He constantly competed with Samaranch. If Samaranch got the largest suite, Nebiolo would never be satisfied with the next largest. Because the IOC had an Olympic anthem, Nebiolo ordered one to be composed immediately for the IAAF. Nebiolo was determined that only he in the world of international sport would measure up to Samaranch.

The vane rivalry between Nebiolo and Samaranch also brought about a number of good things too. 'One result that still remains because of their personal rivalry was the establishment of the Court of Arbitration for Sport, or CAS. This happened when the IAAF was being drawn into ever more legal disputes, most of them related to doping cases. Nebiolo realised that we needed to find a way to avoid repeatedly ending up in costly court cases. I informed him about the Swedish system – *Riksidrottsnämnden* – the Swedish sports tribunal. Thanks to the calibre of its members it maintained an excellent reputation.

'With *Riksidrottsnämnden* as a model, the IAAF decided in 1982 to establish a court of arbitration, the IAAF arbitration panel, as the highest ruling body for disputes within the IAAF. It only took Samaranch a year to follow suit and establish the CAS, which today is internationally recognised as the highest ruling body within sport. The majority of these cases are actually related to doping. CAS is recognised by the Swiss judiciary, and with its Lausanne headquarters, it operates under Swiss legislation.

'Nebiolo was very career- and goal-orientated. Sport was his life and intrigue was the instrument he used. He and Samaranch were very similar. Samaranch was once the Spanish ambassador in Moscow and he was equally power-fixated as Nebiolo. However, instead of intrigue he put his diplomatic capabilities to full effect. That was how he put an end to the escalating number of boycotts and got China back into the Olympic fold in 1984 and South Africa in 1992.

'And which politician would have been able to get North and South Korea to march in under the same banner at the opening ceremony of the Olympics? This happened at the Sydney Olympics in 2000 and in Athens 2004. This act has been a clear indication to the world how the people of Korean peninsula really would like it to be. It was Samaranch's masterpiece.

'Nebiolo was more of a dictator. I had a great deal of controversies with him when he bypassed the council and made decisions on his own accord – decisions we got to find out about from the media. One example of this was when the American sprinter Michael Johnson hadn't qualified for the world championships.

'In one swift move, Nebiolo rewrote the rules so that every defending champion was automatically invited to participate at the following world championships. It was a great idea but it would have been better if Nebiolo had discussed it first with his colleagues on the IAAF council.

'Journalists started ringing me to ask what I thought about the change in rules, but I didn't have a clue what they were talking about. I only found out what Nebiolo had done from them. So stated I publicly that I was completely against this way of deciding things.

'Then Nebiolo asked me, as he always did when he had been criticised or questioned, "Why are you against me?" It was his standard phrase.'

Nebiolo's obsession with Samaranch wasn't just based on his personal vanity. He was also obsessed with the idea of becoming an IOC member. At that time members of the IOC were selected by the president of the IOC, based on the recommendation of retiring IOC members. As Nebiolo wasn't particularly popular back home in Italy, there wasn't much chance that a retiring IOC member would nominate him.

Nebiolo saw one final chance to get into the IOC, and that was via the IAAF. It was natural, he argued, that the president of the largest Olympic federation, the IAAF, should be on the IOC. He courted Samaranch so persistently that in the end, the IOC gave in and created a new rule, the 'Nebiolo Law'.

'I know that the Swedish IOC member Gunnar Ericsson voted against him, which Nebiolo found out about, of course. "Why are you Swedes against me?" he complained to me.'

'Later on, a quota was put on the number of presidents from international sports federations that could become IOC members. The rule stipulated that, without exception, membership of the IOC was to cease at the same time as the member ceased to be president of a federation. Only Nebiolo was permitted to remain in the IOC for life. And that wasn't because he was popular, because he wasn't. It was because he clung on and was feared.'

IT MIGHT BE thought that Primo Nebiolo's way of doing things would have resulted in people questioning his suitability as IAAF president. But the only time his position was seriously threatened was after the world championships were staged in Rome in 1987, and 'the Evangelisti Affair'.

Nebiolo was chairman of the local organising committee of those world championships and, therefore, had ultimate responsibility for its proper conduct.

The long jump was promoted as one of the highlight events of the championships, involving a great battle between the American track superstar, Carl Lewis, and Robert Emmiyan, competing for the Soviet Union. In the event, Italy's Giovanni Evangelisti was awarded the bronze medal after a close contest with another American, Larry Myricks.

But something was not quite right.

Evangelisti jumped first in each round, and in the third round of jumps he moved into third place with 8.19 metres. Myricks overtook the Italian later in the same round with 8.23, and he seemed to have secured the bronze medal when, in the fifth round, the American jumped 8.33.

In to the sixth and final round, and roared on by the Italian fans, Evangelisti produced an excellent effort. The crowd roared when '8.38' was flashed on to the scoreboard – he had done enough to win the bronze medal.

But people who were sitting close to the event saw that the jump had been incorrectly measured.

'Bengt Forsman, a member of the board of the Swedish Sports Confederation, was sitting right in front of the long jump. He came rushing up to me and asked: "Arne, did you see that? It's crazy!" I couldn't believe it when he told me about the incorrect measurement.'

When the suspicions reached the organising committee, they announced that the matter would be investigated.

As the investigation was underway the media began to speculate that Nebiolo was behind the whole thing. The ground began to shake beneath his feet.

'As soon as the investigation was complete, I asked Nebiolo if the IAAF council could be informed of its findings. He said no – because it was in Italian and we wouldn't understand anything. Instead, he offered to appoint his own internal investigation from within the IAAF, with three trustworthy mates.'

The internal investigation resulted in a decision at the IAAF council meeting held in London in April 1988 to withdraw Evangelisti's medal because of the false measurement, while it was maintained that Nebiolo was not involved in any way and had not done anything untoward. But parts of the investigation had been leaked to the media, who in any case had started to carry out their own investigations, using videos of the event and computer analysis which seemed to indicate that Evangelisti had only jumped about 8.15 metres. CONI, the Italian Olympic committee, stepped in with its own investigation.

It really looked like cheating had gone on and that Nebiolo was involved.

In March 1988, CONI's report concluded that Italian athletics federation officials had 'conspired to falsify the measurement of Evangelisti's jump in order to ensure a medal for Italy'. There was even filmed evidence of an official placing a marker in the sand pit *before* Evangelisti's final jump.

'When all this came out, we had an IAAF council meeting in Singapore the following January, where Nebiolo offered some kind of claptrap in his own defence.

'It's an understatement to say that his position was precarious. The only way out was to have the council express its support for him. But he didn't dare to put it to a vote because we'd made it quite clear that we had no confidence in him. After a ballot all we would need to do was call an extraordinary Congress and remove him from office. Nebiolo knew this and he knew he was really in trouble. The claptrap he told us didn't stand scrutiny as an explanation. Publicly, we maintained that we had received a report. That's all.

'But you wouldn't believe it. When the board reconvened the next morning we were told that Nebiolo had informed the world's press that the council had expressed its confidence in him. I immediately said that I wanted it recorded in the minutes that I had never been party to such a decision. I received support from some of my colleagues, including Carl-Olaf Homen, who was on the council as he was president of the European Athletics Association. I also got to see Nebiolo's press release. It was cleverly worded and gave the impression that he had received our full backing.

'What do you call something like this? When I objected, Nebiolo turned pale. He came over to me at the next coffee break. "Arne, come with me," he said, taking me to one side. He started off with his usual phrase. "Arne, why are you against me?" But you could see he was shaken.

'I explained to him that we had not given him our backing and that his statement was wrong. He had lied.

'But this was how he tried to charm his way out of problems he created. Nebiolo rode out the Evangelisti storm but there were certain reprisals which are quite funny in the light of some of the things he had earlier said to me.

'This is how it was. I had stepped down as president of the Swedish athletics association in March 1981. At an IAAF council meeting some time later, Nebiolo took me to one side and asked: "What's happened?"

'What do you mean, what's happened?' I replied.

'"Why have you had to step down as president in Sweden?"' I explained that it's normal in Sweden. I had never imagined being president for more than eight years. Besides, my international assignments were increasing. He scratched his head and after a moment said: "Arne, I will give you a piece of advice. Never give up a position."

'That's how a power-seeker talked. But after the Evangelisti affair, Nebiolo's position as president of FIDAL, Italy's national athletics association, became untenable. Even as the master tactician that he was, he found that prevention was better than the cure. So without warning, he announced that he had so many international assignments that he was leaving the Italian association and he threw a massive party in his own honour. Samaranch and a whole host of dignitaries were invited and along they came, eulogising Nebiolo's fantastic contribution and indispensable position as president of the Italian association. "Never leave a position."'

ARNE WAS AT his cottage on Blidö – an island in the Stockholm archipelago – in the early summer of 1990 when a call came through. It was Nebiolo.

'It was Primo himself who rang. Usually, he let someone else call to show how important he was. "Arne, you better come here," he said.

'"What the hell's happened now?" I wondered.'

The draw for football's World Cup had taken place with the opening match to be played at the new Stadio delle Alpi in Turin – Nebiolo's home city – and the match would be between Sweden and Brazil.

Nebiolo felt that Arne had to be there. It was his instinctive political feeling. '"You are the most senior representative for Swedish sport. And you are my vice-president. You have to sit next to me, otherwise people will wonder what's going on," he told me. But I didn't have the time or inclination. I wanted to stay with my family out in the archipelago. So he put it more clearly: "You had better come; bring the family."

'He was extraordinarily hospitable and pleasant. When I got there with my wife Ulla and one of our sons, we were invited to a reception on the top floor of a ten-storey building where he had his private quarters. The lift went up to his private entrance hall. He showed us out on to the balcony which had an exceptional view over Turin, and then he pointed to a building lower down on the ground. "That's where Agnelli lives," he said. He meant Gianni Agnelli, the head of Fiat, one of Italy's most powerful men and one of the world's leading industrialists.

'Nebiolo was visibly touched that he could look down at Agnelli's home from his own residence. I then understood that there was a good deal of humour behind the mask. Looking back I can see that many times we had a lot of fun together.

BUT NEBIOLO WAS never much fun when it came to Arne's work in anti-doping. 'He didn't like the negative publicity the IAAF got because we continually caught athletes taking performance-enhancing substances. But he recognised that the work had gone too far to be ignored by the time he took over the position of president in 1981. So it was with little support, and up against a certain amount of passive resistance, that I was allowed to carry on, until the Ben Johnson scandal in 1988.'

Nebiolo remained in office throughout the 1990s – 'Never leave a position' – and for someone in his seventies, he continued to travel widely and work long hours. But

Arne could see how he had aged, and when towards the end of the decade Arne noticed Nebiolo suffering from cramp, he attempted to talk to him. He was a physician, after all.

'I remember that we were in Seville for the 1999 world championships. We were staying at the same hotel as usual, the Alfonso XIII. Nebiolo was in a pretty bad way. He was carefully treading water in the pool. Primo himself didn't want to talk to me about it. When I tried to talk to Giovanna, his wife, who both Ulla and I got on very well with, she wouldn't talk about her husband's illness either.'

Within a few months, Primo Nebiolo had died, aged seventy-six.

'I hadn't realised that his illness was so severe. He told me that he went jogging in the swimming pool every morning to build up his strength, but when I thought more about it afterwards, I could see there was evidence that he had started to lose his grip on negotiations.'

Primo Nebiolo left a significant mark on international sport. He had been president of the IAAF for eighteen years, and by the time of his death the organisation had been transformed, both financially and in terms of prestige.

'They say that results matter. The result of Nebiolo's presidency for athletics was outstanding. And personally, I have come to miss him.'

Chapter 8

The Anti-Doping Police and the East German Underworld

THE MAJORITY OF Arne's international anti-doping work is based on his experiences in Sweden. Before he put his knowledge and experience to use internationally, he had wanted to 'put his own house in order'. However, his work in Sweden was just as much about finding the right way forward generally, as he sought strategies that would work.

A cornerstone in the work against doping is testing for drugs. But it was recognised early on that it was not enough just to test for drugs during competitions. It was soon obvious that athletes just had to stop taking their anabolic steroids in time for the competition. With the testing that was available at competitions in the late 1970s and 1980s, it was impossible to detect drug-use if athletes stopped taking drugs ahead of a tested event. Athletes and their coaches had enough medical knowledge to know when they would need to stop in order not to fail a drugs test – what became known as 'clearance time'. The few that still tested positive at that time had simply miscalculated.

But how far was it possible to go in order to control the athletes outside of competition without encroaching upon their privacy and integrity? It was a question Arne asked himself as early as the end of the 1970s.

'I needed to know if it was legally possible to test athletes at any time for the use of performance-enhancing drugs. Was it possible for us to just turn up and take a drug test? To turn up at their work or at their home and just ask for a urine sample for analysis? The answers that I received from lawyers suggested that it was possible to do that without encroaching upon the athletes' rights.'

It was actually a clear cut case. The legal experts told Arne that when an athlete joins a sports club which falls under the jurisdiction of the Swedish Sports Confederation, then they fall subject to the rules and regulations of the Confederation. So if these rules stipulate that a member can be required to provide a urine sample for testing, at any time and anywhere, then it is deemed that the athlete has accepted these terms when he or she became a member of the club.

'It's perfectly possible to refuse to provide a sample, but in doing so you step outside the rules and regulations. After all, it's not obligatory to be a member of a sports club.

'Legally, it seemed as clear as daylight. As soon as the Swedish Sports Confederation amended its rules and regulations at the end of the 1970s, it became possible to require a urine sample from an athlete at any time. It came to be known as "out-of-competition testing" – or OOC tests. They were first carried out in Sweden in 1982.'

OOC TESTS WOULD become the most important tool in the work to combat doping, but they were initially met with opposition. Just because Swedish legal experts interpreted the rules and regulations in favour of an OOC testing programme, it wasn't taken for granted that it would be interpreted in the same way outside Sweden. Work got underway in the Nordic countries to convince the rest of the world that the tests were both legal and necessary. 'Norway had the same legal interpretation as we did, and very soon Finland and Denmark came on board. In 1983, we signed a "Nordic Convention" that made all Nordic athletes subject to the OOC tests.'

This was the first international anti-doping convention, a model that the present IOC president, Jacques Rogge, has referred to as a predecessor of the World Anti-Doping Agency, that was formed in the twenty-first century.

'You would have thought that the work would now be easier and that the other countries would follow suit just because the Nordic countries had cleared the way. But it wasn't like that at all. My West German colleague, Manfred Donike, who was on the medical committee at both the IOC and IAAF, had been working with the issue of performance-enhancing drugs as long as I had, if not longer. He considered that an OOC testing programme would be completely unthinkable in West Germany. It would be interpreted as an insult to people's freedoms. The Germans would eventually be forced to think again when they had to deal with the East German problem after unification.'

The East Germans were, of course, invited to join the Nordic Convention. Their answer, however, was expected: 'We'd be happy to join as long as the Soviet Union and United States do likewise.'

International opposition to OOC testing was far reaching, even though the system proved to work well in the Nordic countries. There was no lack of interest in it.

'In 1988, we arranged an international anti-doping conference in Borlänge in Sweden which we called "Out of Competition Doping Controls". The response was massive and, without exception, positive. Many delegates, however, felt that it would encroach upon the privacy and freedoms of the athletes. Besides, some felt it would be impossible to find and train all the doping control officers necessary to carry out testing not just at competitions, but all year round.'

The Nordic experience suggested the exact opposite. The initiative got a massive response, particularly from people working within the healthcare sector. Through recruitment, courses and training days, slowly but surely a network of competent individuals who could carry out drug tests was built up by the Swedish Sports Confederation's anti-doping commission, led by Arne. They were known as the 'anti-doping police' by some people.

'I've heard about some early OCC tests where it only took the inspector to turn up at training for the athletes to scuttle away through the doors and windows or hide inside gym equipment, like a vaulting box, or behind the curtains. That's what it looked like in the beginning.

'Nowadays there's a completely different understanding of the work that's being done.'

IT TOOK THE Ben Johnson scandal in 1988 for international opposition to OOC tests to finally melt away. With Arne working from his position within the IAAF, it was at the federation's congress in Barcelona in 1989 that rules were introduced which enabled unannounced drug testing to be implemented worldwide.

And with that, the next problem was encountered. How could officials know where athletes would be at any point in time? 'We started out quite gently, asking the individual associations from each country to take care of the reporting, but we felt that some weren't particularly interested in the matter. So a rule was written in, making athletes responsible for notifying us where they were. But, quite simply, it didn't work. For the 1993 world championships in Stuttgart, Primo Nebiolo announced that a Mercedes would go to each of the gold medallists. That was the beginning of the massive sums of money which are today handed out in prize money, but at the time we realised we could make the most of this. It was decided that anyone who didn't undergo at least two OOC tests per year would not be entitled to receive prize money.

'Some athletes were convinced by this and turned in details of their whereabouts, but the system didn't quite work perfectly yet. In later years, many athletes didn't receive their prize money because they hadn't been available for OOC testing, but that in itself didn't cause many protests.

'I'm convinced that these athletes were compensated at the time by their national federations. So we were forced to tighten the rules even more. In 2003, a rule was introduced which stipulated that an athlete could be punished if he or she turned in false details of their whereabouts, both to their national federation or to the IAAF.

'It was really only at this point that it became possible to carry out truly random drug testing. If an athlete wasn't to be found at the place they had given on their "whereabouts" form, it was reported immediately. If it happened again, then the matter was taken to a higher level and duly noted as a missed test. If the doping control officer tries to reach the athlete to take a sample and fails a third time, the missed test is regarded just the same as a positive drug tests.

'By 2004, the requirement for athletes to declare their whereabouts was introduced into the WADA code, and is applied to competitors in all sports. It's even being discussed, quite seriously, whether elite athletes should be forced to be tagged with a microchip so that they can always be tracked, no matter where they are. It's a controversial suggestion, but there's been a positive response by elite Swedish athletes.'

Respect for the integrity of the OOC testing programme did not come automatically.

Drug tests for the IAAF were handled by a Swedish private company called International Doping Tests and Management (IDTM). One day in the middle of the 1990s, Primo Nebiolo, when president of the IAAF, telephoned Arne.

'I was at my summerhouse. It was Primo's assistant who called. When he came to the phone he sounded upset, angry even. "Arne," he said, "an Italian journalist has told me that IDTM have sent people to Italy and carried out doping tests on Italian runners right in the middle of their training without informing me. This is completely unacceptable. How has this happened? What am I to say to the journalists who are ringing? You must explain yourself!"

'"Listen Primo," I answered. "That's the whole point. No one is to be informed beforehand. Only IDTM is to know who is to be tested and when. That's what you should have told the journalists. You would have then demonstrated how trustworthy our system is. I didn't know that IDTM was going to carry out doping tests in Italy, and we should both be happy that we don't. It shows that our system works."

'Primo wanted to control everything. He was completely behind the OOC tests, but when IDTM turned their attention to Italy, he thought immediately that it was some kind of conspiracy against his country. "Why are you against me and my country?"

'It was good that I got the opportunity to explain to my boss, the president of the federation, how the system was intended to work, that the whole idea was that the test would be given without any prior warning to anyone. Primo changed tack completely during the course of our conversation, saying: "That's great, Arne. Interesting. Really good. Thank you. Goodbye, then."'

THE IAAF's WORK in setting up lasting rules and regulations concerning doping tests did not cease just because OOC tests were introduced. A number of legal challenges were raised. Evidence in a doping case needed to stand up legally in the highest court in the land. This meant that drug tests needed to be better organised and clearly impartial.

'We discussed the issue of whether doping control officers should test athletes who shared the same nationality as them. Wouldn't it affect their credibility if they did? There were rumours that certain agreements had been made between doping control officers and athletes, and that certainly wasn't very good. The same applied to the accredited laboratories that were to carry out the analysis of urine samples. Of course, all tests are anonymous, but in spite of this, several serious challenges occurred.

'The first concerned the laboratory in Rome in 1998. The IOC's medical committee had noted that the Rome lab noticeably reported very few detected cases of steroid-use. Italy's football association had long bragged about its massive testing programme. The tests were sent to the Rome lab, but it turned out that they were never analysed for steroids. This was a conscious decision, of course.

'The head of the lab was fired, along with the entire staff. The lab was stripped of its accreditation and was shut down. Even more heads would roll. The lab was owned by CONI, the Italian Olympic committee and one of the world's richest. The committee lost all its privileges and its chairman was forced to resign. Later, the laboratory reopened under new leadership and has since worked well, including testing for the Turin Winter Olympics in 2006.

'On another occasion it was the Moscow laboratory which was caught. It was after a test had been sent there from the Ukraine. They reported that it was negative, which was good, but the problem was that the Moscow lab hadn't analysed it but sent the test on to another lab. The Moscow lab also had to change management and a new head was appointed.'

The next big issue to be tackled was impartiality. There could be absolutely no hint of a conflict of interests or conflict of loyalties. 'After WADA was established in 1999, it was my wish that the agency should take over responsibility for the IAAF's international OOC tests. This would guarantee impartiality. But the organisation never received sufficient funds. Today, WADA only takes care of the OOC tests in certain countries and within certain sports where anti-doping controls wouldn't otherwise take place. WADA's main role is to monitor and co-ordinate the anti-doping activities that are run globally, set up anti-doping units where there aren't very many or none at all, as well as ensure that the code, the World Anti-Doping Code, which WADA has produced, is respected.

'The IAAF has handed over the running of anti-doping tests to IDTM. It was started by a Swede, Staffan Sahlström, who was connected to the Swedish Sports Confederation during the 1970s and 1980s and helped me build up the Swedish anti-doping organisation which came to be a model for the rest of the world.

'In 1991, he started a business that carried out drug tests on personnel working on oil tankers. It was after the environmental disaster that occurred when the oil tanker Exxon Valdez ran aground just off the coast of Alaska and leaked 260,000 barrels of oil, which destroyed a massive nature reserve. It turned out that the captain had been under the influence of alcohol. With his experience of anti-doping work, Staffan Sahlström could build up a control company to monitor this kind of problem.'

IDTM is nowadays under contract to WADA, the IAAF and many other sporting organisations. They partly handle the taking of doping tests, and also ensure that the tests are securely analysed by accredited laboratories. The transporting of drug tests is carried out with what is known as a 'chain of custody'. IDTM has, since its inception, built up its own network by recruiting, training and qualifying doping control officers in eighty or so countries.

Their headquarters are on the island of Lidingö in Stockholm, with a small team of staff, but around the world they have more than 250 doping control officers contracted to work for them. IDTM carries out more than 5,000 random, out-of-competition drug tests each year and another 3,000 or more tests at competitions. In addition to this, the company also carries out more than 2,500 blood tests on athletes each year.

Although it may seem a bit strange, IDTM works without any kind of competitor. Only a few similar companies have been established. There is one in Germany that provides national tests; there is also a small company serving college sport in the United States. The Association of National Anti-Doping Agencies (ANADO) formed a test organization a few years ago but it does not seem to have been particularly active.

The fact that IDTM is unique in its field isn't without problems. 'When I said several years ago that IDTM is the only organisation that is competent to reliably carry out random drug testing on a global scale, I was accused of having a particular interest in IDTM. There was, among other things, an article in *L'Equipe* in France which spread the rumour. I understand where they were coming from. Early on, Staffan Sahlström approached me and offered me the opportunity to become a part-owner as well as board member of the company. I realised at the time that it would be impossible, so I declined.

'I have never had, and will never have, any personal interests in a company that is likely to clash with my work in sport.'

WORK TO COMBAT the use of drugs in sport was, for many years, complicated by the Cold War. And among the communist countries, athletes from East Germany presented a particular problem. From the mid-1960s, East German competitors dominated international athletics and swimming, as well as several other sports. They won 350 gold medals. Some of the world records they set still stand today. Outside the sports arenas, they behaved in an exemplary manner within an international context, which made them well-liked by both sports leaders and their fellow competitors.

The results they achieved were widely admired. There was uncritical admiration among some journalists and sports leaders, who travelled to East Germany and were impressed by the athlete recruitment and training that they saw.

But others suspected that something wasn't quite as it should be. It was noticed how East German women athletes were extraordinarily muscular and often had facial hair, acne and deep voices. Their female bodies were visibly marked by male hormones. When confronted by the accusation that his women swimmers had uncharacteristically deep voices, one East German swimming coach dismissed all suspicions with what would become remembered as a classic quote: 'Our girls are here to swim, not to sing.'

Then, on a Sunday morning in November 1990, Arne received another important telephone call. 'It was from my East German colleague from the IAAF's medical committee, Manfred Hoeppner. It was just after the reunification of Germany. He had given an interview to a German news magazine, I think it was *Stern*, and he had just received the article for inspection before it went to print. "I've laid all my cards on the table," he told me. "I reveal in the article the systematic doping programme that has existed in East Germany for decades. I want you to be the first to know."

'It didn't come as a surprise to me that East Germany had had a doping programme to achieve their results. The whole world had suspected that to be the case: we'd just lacked any evidence. Hoeppner answered all my questions frankly during the conversation.

'When he finally asked me if I thought he would be able to keep his place on the IAAF's medical committee after this revelation, I answered equally frankly: I didn't think so.

'Soon after that, we accepted his resignation.'

You have to ask yourself what makes a particular country maintain a state-run, systematic doping programme? 'I remember that Sweden won an international match in athletics against East Germany in Leipzig in 1961. East Germany still hadn't recovered from the war. It was a second-rate country when it came to sport. I learned from Hoeppner that East Germany used sport as a means to gain recognition. Maybe that was one reason: that East Germany wanted to assert itself and win recognition both in terms of the international community and the eye of the general public.'

The strategy was both thorough and well-carried out. 'They were seeking success within a sporting context in general and at the Olympic Games in particular. Athletics and swimming were considered the greatest sports, and after analysing the situation it was decided that they would concentrate on the women's events. They were not as developed as men's events and anabolic steroids can enhance the performances of women much more than men. So they launched a campaign to recruit new talents. The recruits' genetic condition was examined. Their parenthood was analysed along with their social background. And, last but not least, East Germany developed its very own steroid, known as Turinabol, in "little blue pills' although it was available as an injectable, too.'

Turinabol was manufactured by Jenapharm, East Germany's state pharmaceutical company. 'Sure, we had ways to analyse this anabolic steroid, too. It was just that the doping programme in East Germany was so well-controlled that the athletes were always "clean" ahead of competitions where doping tests would be carried out.'

But even the well-organised East Germans miscalculated their schedule occasionally. The shot putter Ilona

Slupianek, among others, failed two drugs tests. The West could only guess that these discoveries were just the top of an iceberg.

'The East German doping programme was carefully tested and governed from the very top. At the same time they categorically denied what was going on. It was even the case that Hoeppner, on the IAAF's medical committee under me, and thus a part of the anti-doping work of the 1970s and 1980s was part of the cover up. His duties included handling the East German anti-doping programme, without us knowing about his role.

'East Germany even had its very own accredited doping laboratory in Kreischa, which of course was just a part of the sophisticated cheating apparatus that their system set up. The whole thing was just a massive sham. I have seen Dr Hoeppner standing there, teaching doping control officers at an IAAF workshop in Barcelona, answering questions and pretending to be engaged in the anti-doping movement.

'And the head of the Kreischa laboratory, Clausnitzer, a member of the IOC's medical committee, always quick to criticise other laboratories for flawed analyses. But never once did his lab report a positive case of doping among East German athletes.

'Of course, he was fired soon after the fall of the Berlin Wall. I met him a few times and found him to be a very pleasant person and easy to chat to. But the same applied to most of them in East Germany, because it was part of their strategy: be nice and polite.'

In East Germany, officials would speak of their 'medical support programme' for their athletes. In the West, this was understood as a programme aimed at helping competing athletes handle the massive strain they were put under, both mentally and physically, as if it was something to prevent injuries.

'Once, during one of his visits to Stockholm, I invited Hoeppner to my home. We sat in the sauna and had just started talking about the medical programme in East Germany. I was discussing different types of monitoring, ways you could guard against injury, and how you could follow-up on those athletes that had been injured.

'Then Hoeppner let something slip. He said: "Sometimes you need to give them certain medication too."

'"Which medication?" I asked, but quickly he recovered and kept quiet. But I continued, explaining that if the strain was now so immense that athletes needed to take medication to be able to continue, then we doctors needed to make sure that they weren't exposed to so much stress that made them ill. Hoeppner conceded the point.

'When, a year later, he telephoned me and told me about the article in *Stern*, he said in confidence that he had only ever doubted the East German doping system and its moral and medical tenability on just one occasion – in the sauna at my place.'

EAST GERMANY'S STATE doping programme robbed generations of international sportsmen and women of the opportunity to participate in honest competition. But it also forced East Germany's own competitors to pay an awful price for their success. 'We could see how people were changed by the medication they were forced to take. I think it's strange that there's never been any scientific research on what consequences the East German phenomenon had on the individuals involved, and society as a whole.

'I know that the German couple Brigitte Berendonk and Werner Franke revealed some of what went on in East Germany after Brigitte left the country. Her account is based on her own experiences and also documents from the Stasi, the East German secret police, and tells what she and her husband went through after the Berlin Wall came down.

'Brigitte's book, *Doping Dokumente,* is an important document, but there still isn't a systematic and scientific analysis of the effect of doping on humans and society, on a whole nation.

'My colleague, doping researcher Professor Manfred Donike, from Cologne in western Germany, believed it was time for the Germans to look forward, but I still think that it is necessary to document the phenomena, both from a social and medical viewpoint. It was a gigantic experiment that went on, where people were selected and put into training and then fed steroids. Today many of them are in their fifties and sixties. It's almost too late to hear what they have to say. Some have spoken out, for example the former sprinter Ines Geipel, who I met in a debate in Berlin in 2008. But there are still many questions that are to be answered.

'The two words that best sum up this era are "Cold War". And it was East Germany that started this Cold War in sport. The great Cold War that raged between East and West was already established, but it was carried into the sports arena, where the main weapon was those little blue pills from Jenapharm, the state pharmaceutical company – East Germany's anabolic steroids.'

Sport's Cold War was fought on all levels. At one point, the Soviet Union and United States entered into an agreement that was intended as a version of the Nordic convention that had been so successful. But Arne viewed the American–Soviet agreement as a pure diversion, intended to show goodwill and an intention to stop drug-use, when in reality both countries had everything to hide and cover-up. The agreement allowed for mutual doping controls, but in fact it proved to be little more than a public relations stunt, something that existed on paper but not in reality through any actions.

Once the Cold War was over between the politicians and the Iron Curtain came down, massive stocks of anabolic steroids were found in Russia. It was these that were later smuggled to Sweden under the name 'Russian Fives', not because they cost five kronor, but because they were five milligram doses.

Chapter 9

Before and After WADA

BY THE END of the 1990s, the work against doping was in a stronger position than ever before. Doping in sport had been recognised as a problem both nationally in Sweden and internationally. Measures had been instigated to get the better of it: the number of doping tests had increased, analysis methods refined, the rules and regulations had been made legally secure. With the Cold War over between the Eastern bloc and the West, there was improved co-operation between sporting bodies, too.

Yet the anti-doping movement still had new challenges to face.

The problem now facing Arne and his colleagues was partly a result of the success they had achieved. Country after country, sport after sport, and federation after federation had introduced their own regulations. Different sports' anti-doping rules sometimes conflicted. Different sports or different countries might dish out different punishments or reach different judgements for similar offences. The co-ordinated regulations across all sports found in Sweden were absent on an international level. Sometimes, conflicts arose between the national and international regulations.

The whole situation seemed to be heading for a problem. If, for example, the Swedish cycling federation had a doping case to take care of, they had to follow both the Swedish national rules and those of the International Cycling Union. The national rules were often more stringent than the rules of the international governing body. Swedish sportsmen and women often found themselves having to accept regulations in Sweden where the penalties were much harsher than those applied in the rest of the world.

There was also uncertainty over who had the responsibility for carrying out the work against doping. The world governing body for athletics, the IAAF, had pushed the matter from the start, so that by the end of the 1990s, track and field accounted for sixty per cent of all out-of-competition tests carried out in the world of sport. Next was swimming, which conducted twenty per cent of the OOC tests. The remaining twenty per cent of tests were conducted by a handful of other sports, but most international federations didn't have any OOC tests at all. Some federations didn't even have rules that allowed for such tests to be carried out.

The same applied to the majority of countries around the world. From the early 1980s, the Nordic region had co-ordinated OOC tests and strict regulations. But nearly twenty years later, Sweden, Finland, Norway and Denmark remained as merely a shining example of how these matters should be handled, with the rest of the world only adopting the policies piecemeal and slowly.

There was one case in the mid-1990s when an Asian woman sprinter was found to have used anabolic steroids after failing an OOC test carried out by the IAAF. But the IAAF could not penalise the athlete because there were simply no rules in her country that allowed for this type of doping control. Similarly, the case of world sprint champion Katrin Krabbe had to be dismissed. She and two colleagues had given identical urine samples at an out-of-competition test while training in South Africa in January 1992, but their cases could not be pursued in the absence of rules in Germany that would allow such testing

Even just in athletics, the contradictory and unclear regulations around the world resulted too often in the IAAF ending up in legal disputes over its high-profile 'war against doping'. It was easy for lawyers to find contradictions and inconsistencies in the rules of sport, and the court cases were time-consuming and expensive.

'The whole thing was unacceptable. It didn't work any more, I had been nagging IOC President Samaranch for ages, telling him we in the world of athletics were having a tough time handling the anti-doping work on our own.'

What was needed was an independent anti-doping organisation supported by the entire sporting world and operating under international law. Arne persuaded Primo Nebiolo, the IAAF president, to come on board. And on the IAAF's initiative, the International Olympic Committee eventually took action.

There were several good reasons for the IOC to pay attention at the end of the 1990s. First was the scandal over the IOC-accredited anti-doping laboratory in Rome in 1998. Another was the scandal at the Tour de France the same year. Under the jurisdiction of the French anti-doping laws, the police carried out a number of raids on the hotel bedrooms of the competing cyclists. After someone tipped off the police, the crackdown targeted the Festina team. The informant was right.

The Tour is France's and cycling's greatest annual sporting event. Indeed, it is one of the world's great annual sporting events. The Festina Affair generated a massive controversy, with headlines on the pack pages, and front pages, around the world. Yet if the whole thing had been handled by the International Cycling Union, the cyclists and team staff concerned, instead of facing criminal charges from the French police, might have only had to pay a few minor fines.

A third reason for the IOC's action was Samaranch himself. When the call for an independent anti-doping organisation began to be heard, he misjudged the situation and made a number of sloppy and unfortunate statements. On one occasion, Samaranch said that substances which were not dangerous to a competitor's health although they could improve performance ought to be allowed.

'The Rome affair was one incitement; the police raid on the Tour de France another, and Samaranch's statements a third. It was clear the time was right.'

The outcome was the World Anti-Doping Agency, or WADA.

'WADA is still relatively new. There were many more people than just me who contributed to it being created. In his memoir, Dick Pound, the former Canadian swimmer and the first WADA president, claims that it was he who pointed out to Samaranch that the situation was untenable. I can live with that.

'But Pound had not been working in anti-doping before WADA was created and I believe that it was the IAAF's experiences and pressure from Nebiolo that really put it on its way. And I was behind both of these moves.'

FOLLOWING PRELIMINARY MEETINGS, the IOC summoned all the sports federations and national Olympic committees to a world conference about doping in sport in Lausanne at the beginning of February 1999. Also invited were government representatives from around the world.

'It was something completely new to see Samaranch and Nebiolo working towards the same goal. It had never happened before. It was known that they weren't the best of friends.'

Europe was well represented and the Swedish government minister responsible attended along with her Nordic colleagues. After a series of discussions, the Olympic movement and the political establishment decided to join forces.

The conference delivered the 'Lausanne Declaration', which called for the establishment of an independent international anti-doping agency whose purpose was to co-ordinate the rules and activities against doping in sport. This was to be fully operational by the time of the Sydney Olympic Games the following year. Another conference was held in November 1999 when representatives of the Olympic movement and public authorities agreed upon some fundamental details so that WADA could be founded formally.

The agency was to be half-financed by the IOC and half by international governments. This was no problem for the IOC, but governments found it difficult to find ways to finance an organisation like WADA and to agree on how much each of them should contribute. The delay in securing the public funding formula meant that WADA started with a rather limited budget, something which, happily, was resolved before too long.

Today, WADA receives something in the region of US$25 million per year, of which around twenty-five per cent goes towards research. 'That part is used to improve existing methods of analysis and to develop testing methods, as new

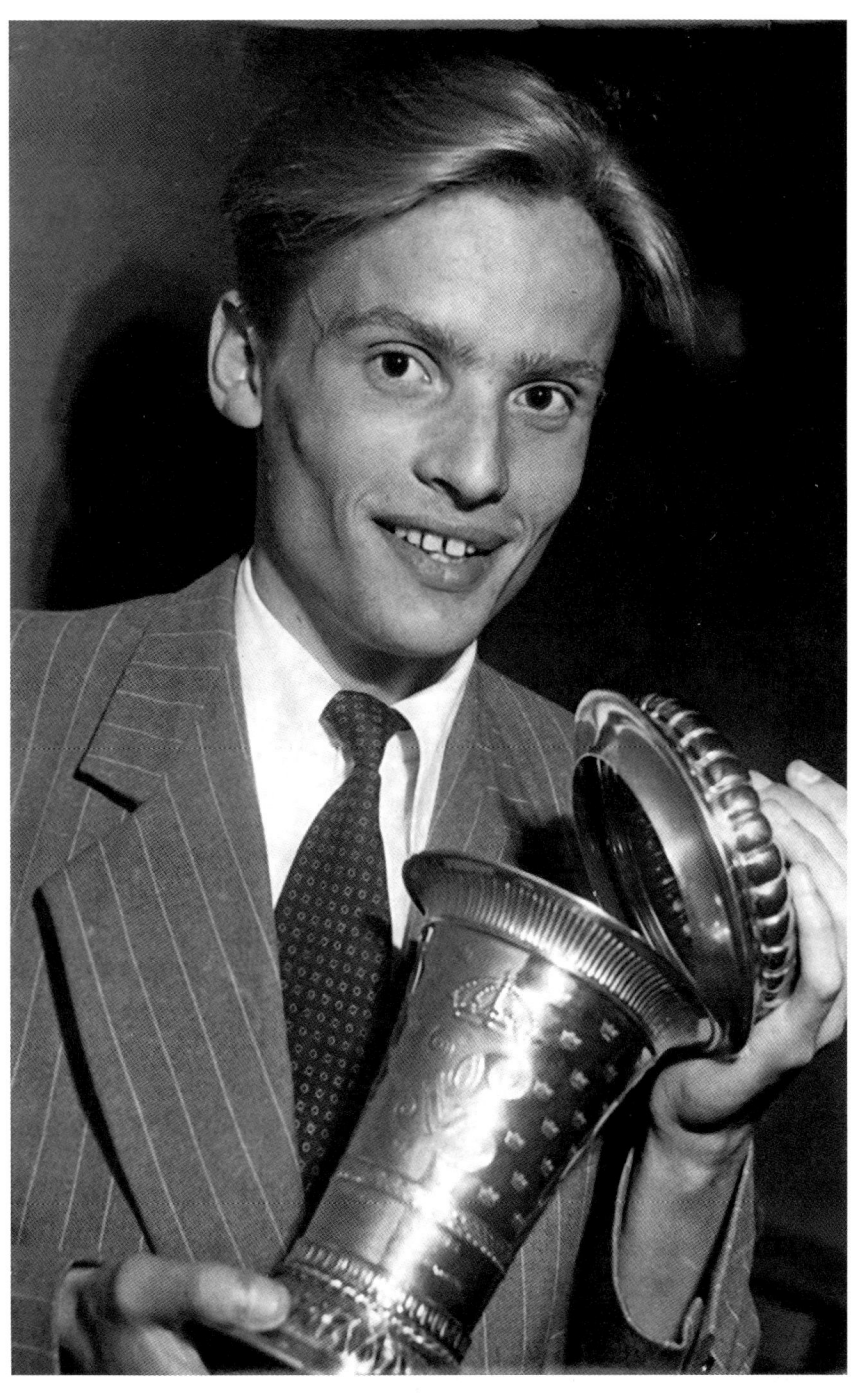

Arne with the King's Cup after triumphs in the National Autumn School Athletics Games of 1949.

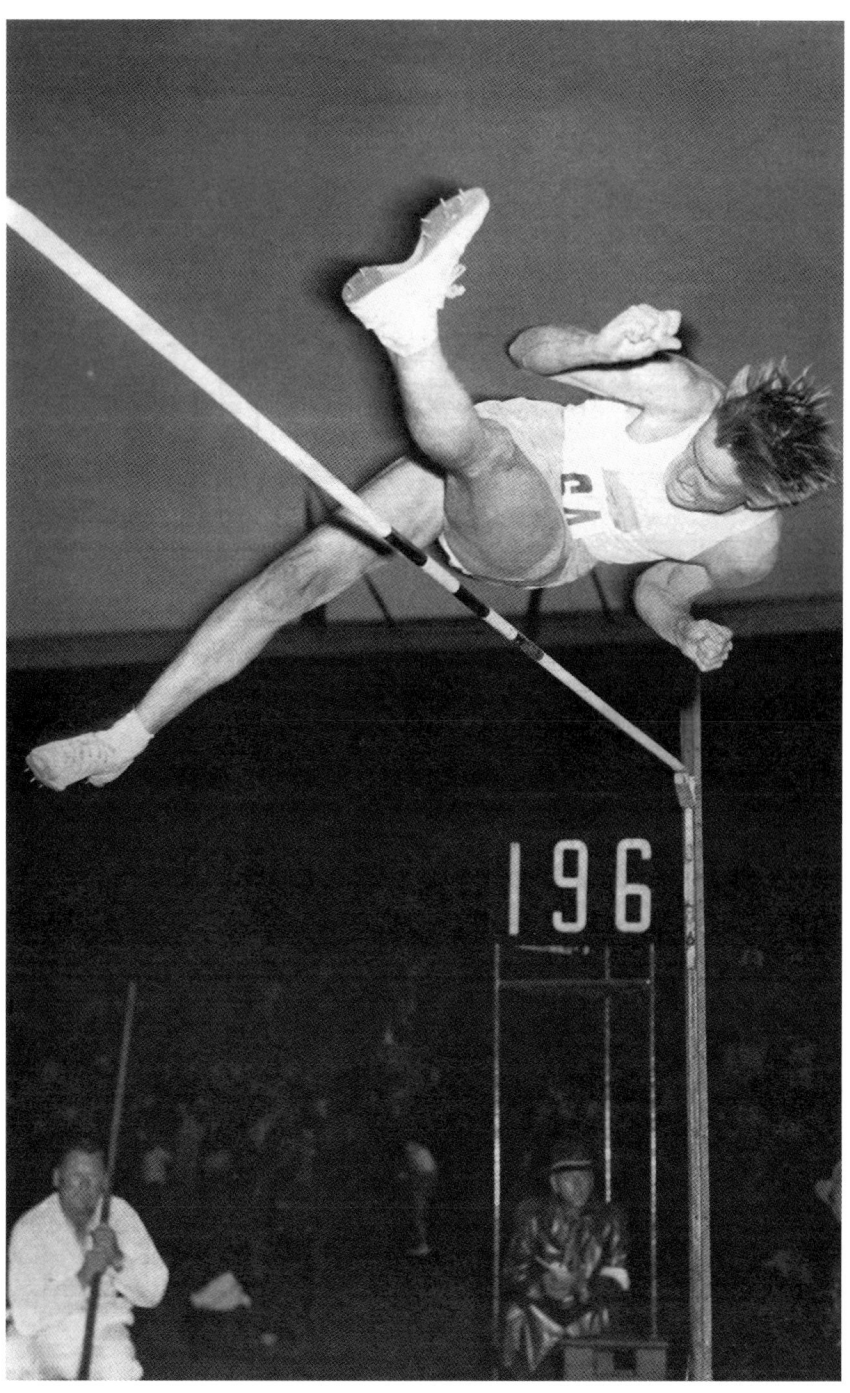

Arne wins the high jump in the match against Germany in the Stockholm Stadium in 1951 by clearing 1.96m.

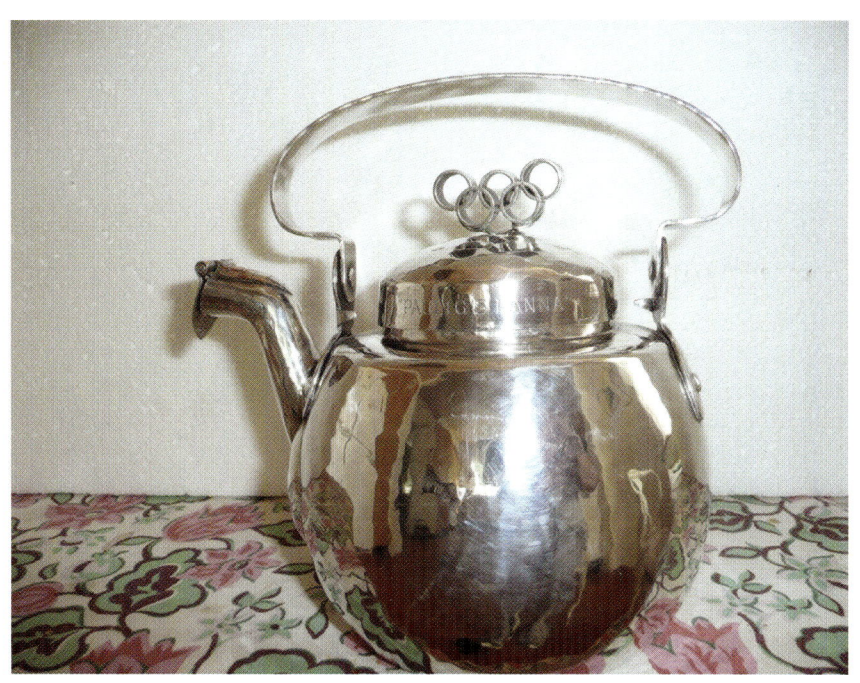

Paulig's coffee pot awarded for Arne's performance in the Finnkampen in Finland.

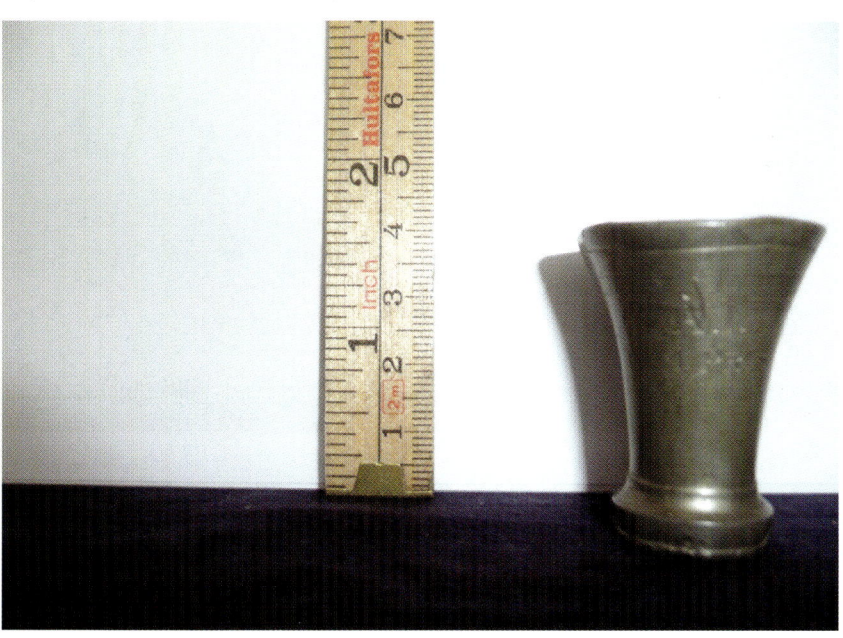

The Kabom Trophy, awarded to Arne as the top Swedish athlete when Sweden beat Germany in 1951.

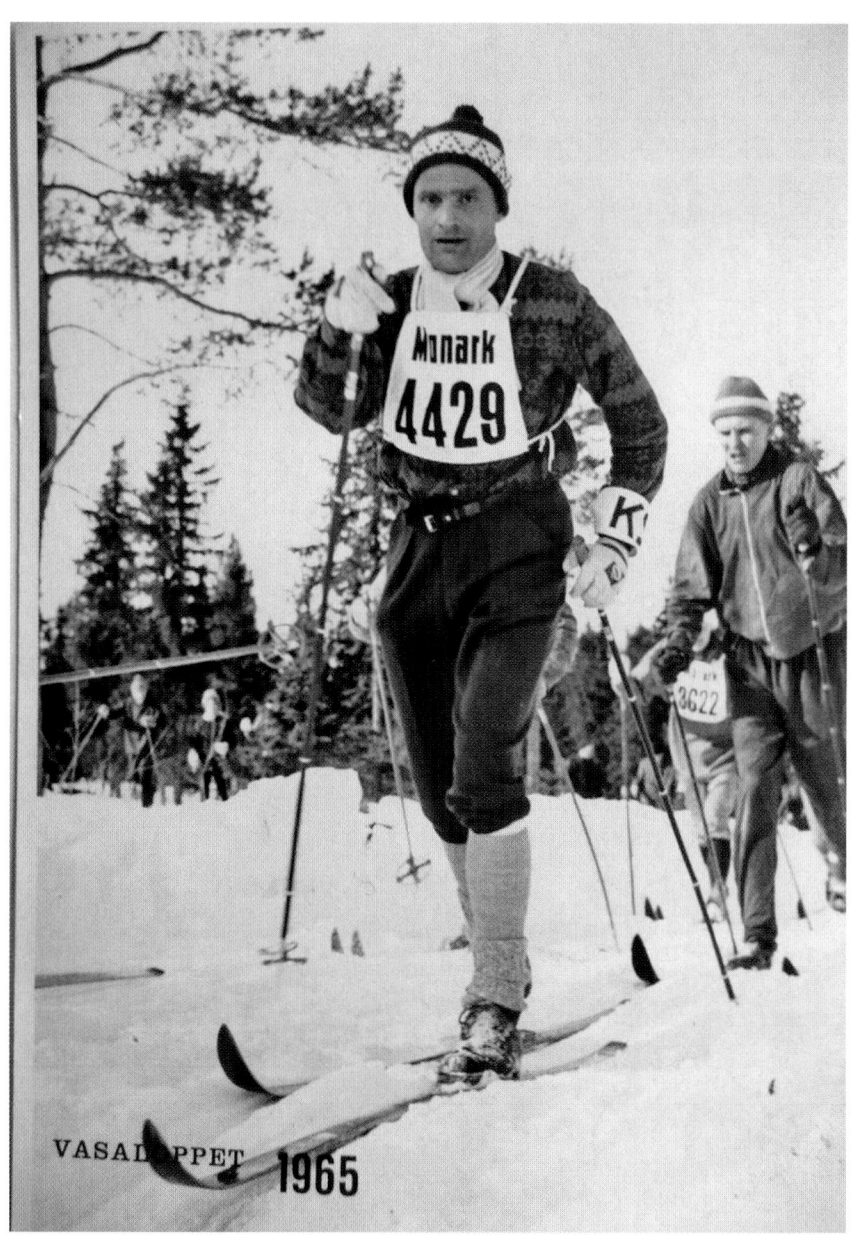

Arne competing in the Vasaloppet in 1965, a 90km
cross country ski race in Sweden.

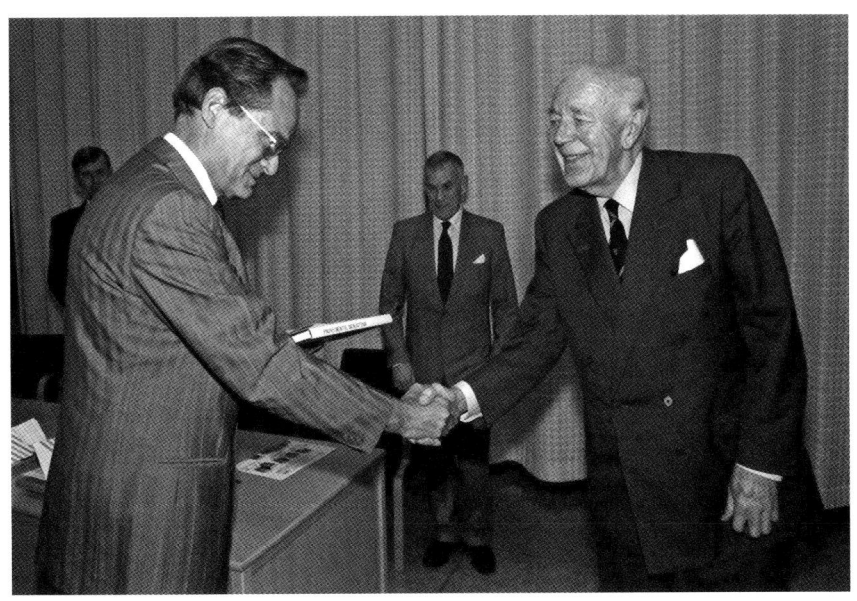

*Prince Bertil hands over the Award named 'The Prince's Medal'
at the annual meeting of the Swedish Association for the
Promotion of Sports in 1990.*

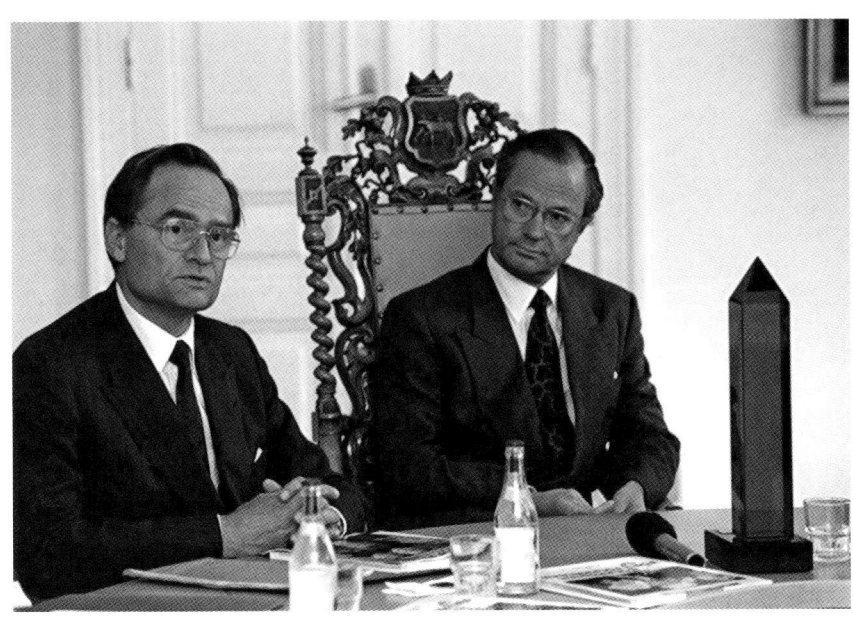

*Together with his Majesty the King at the celebration at the residence of
Östersund in the early nineties because of the victory of the
region of Östersund in the Cancer Society's National Walk.*

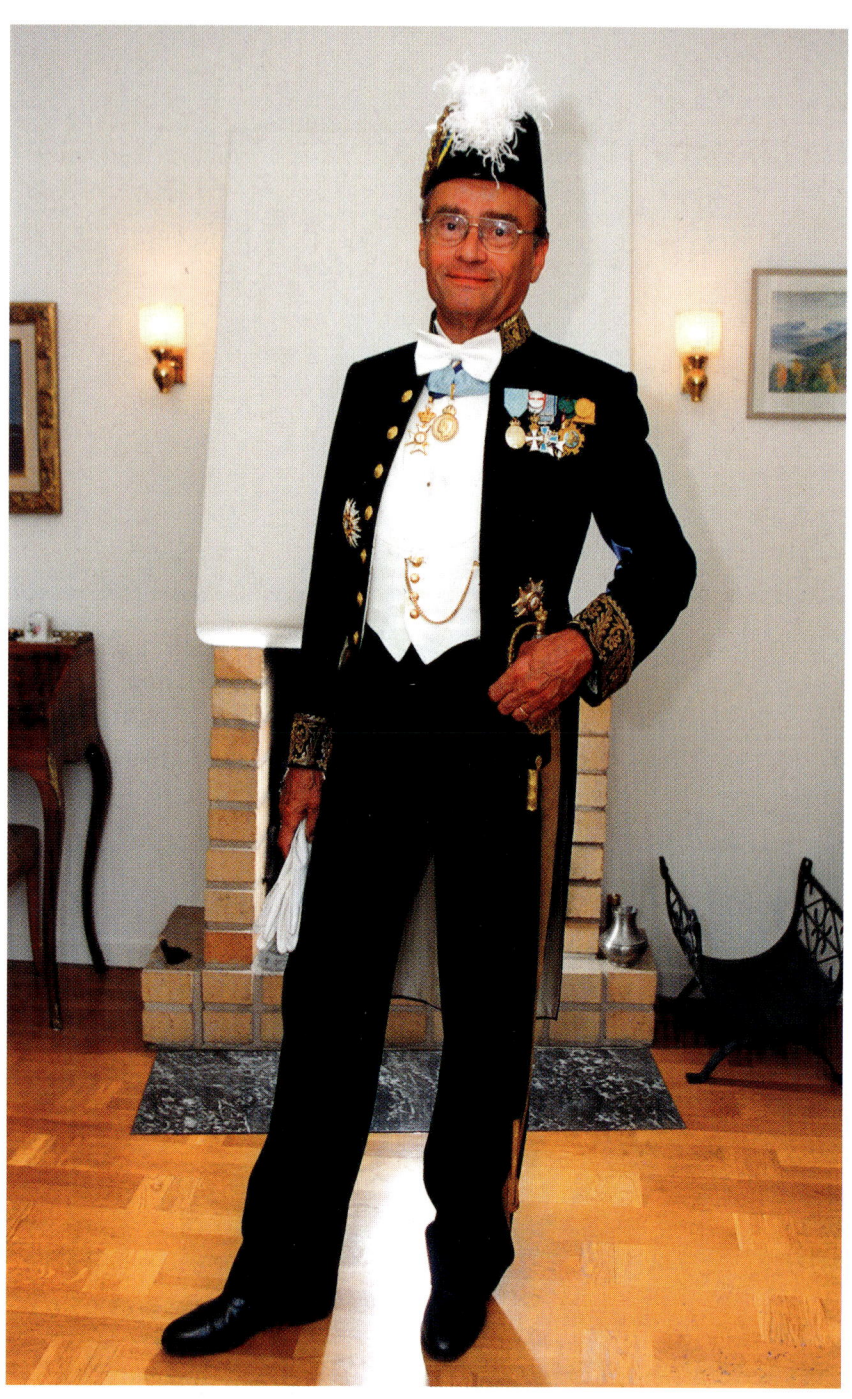

The uniform of the Lord-in-waiting.

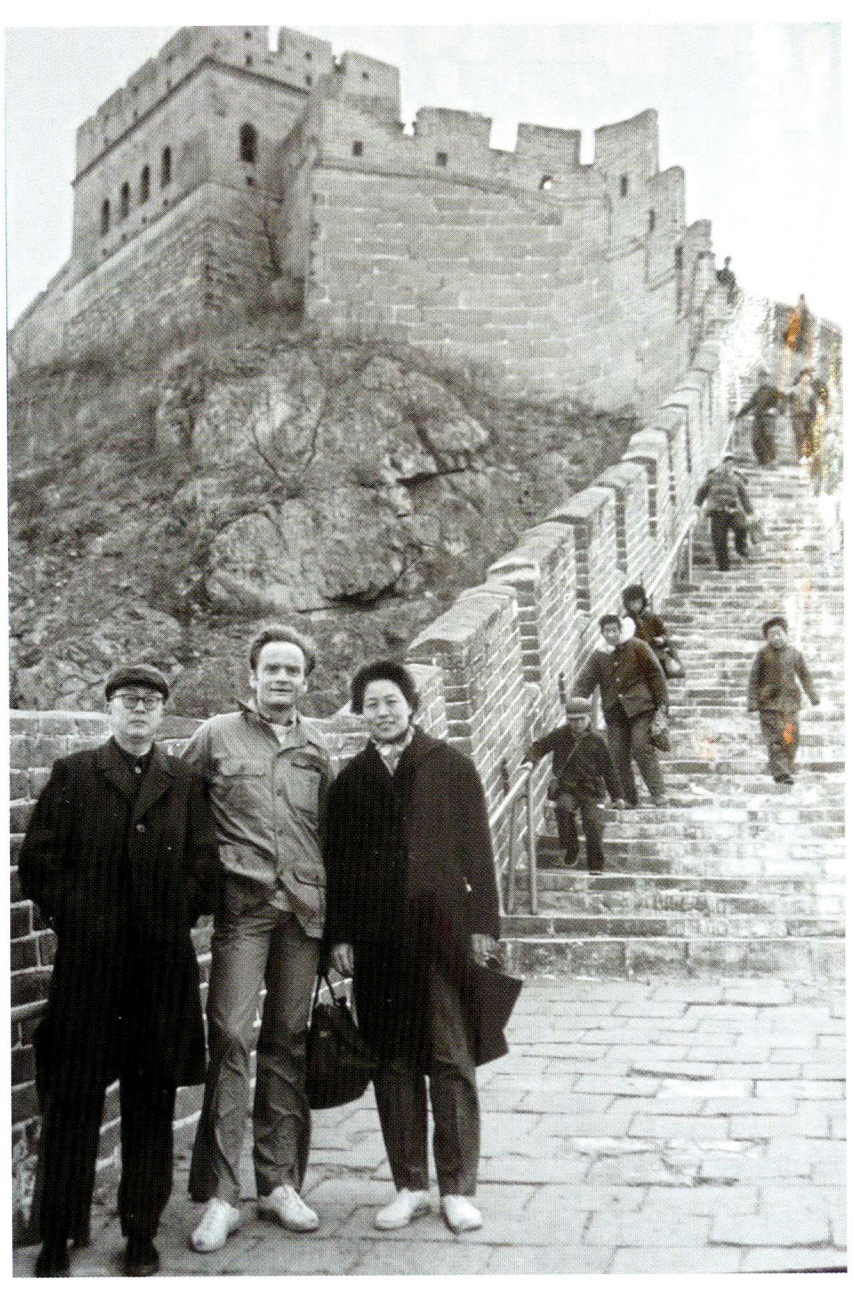

Arne at the Great Wall outside Bejing in 1978 together with his Chinese 'minder' (in those days people were not allowed to travel around in China on their own). On his left is Chen Feng-jung who set a new women's high jump world record in 1957 of 1.77m.

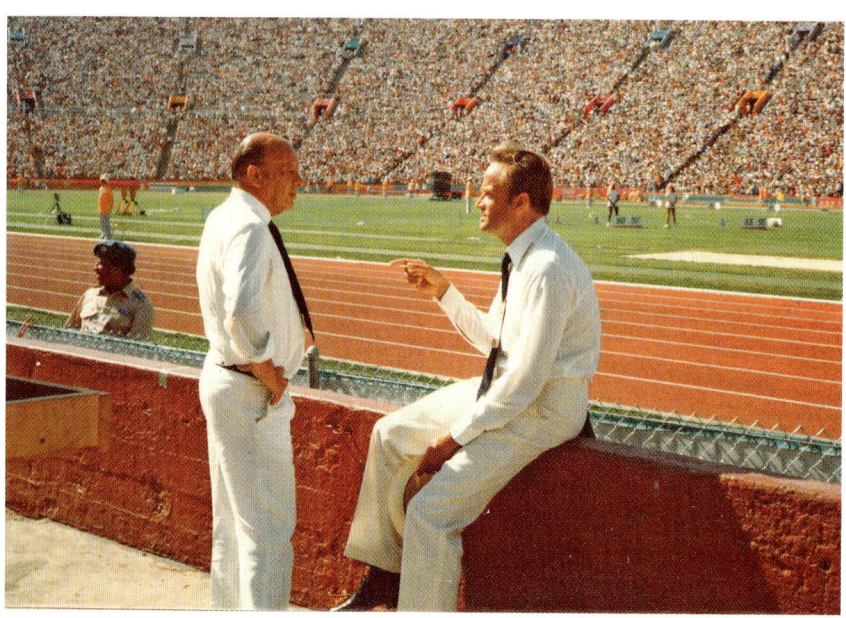

Arne and IAAF president Primo Nebiolo discuss the Martti Vainio Case in the Olympic Stadium in Los Angeles 1984.

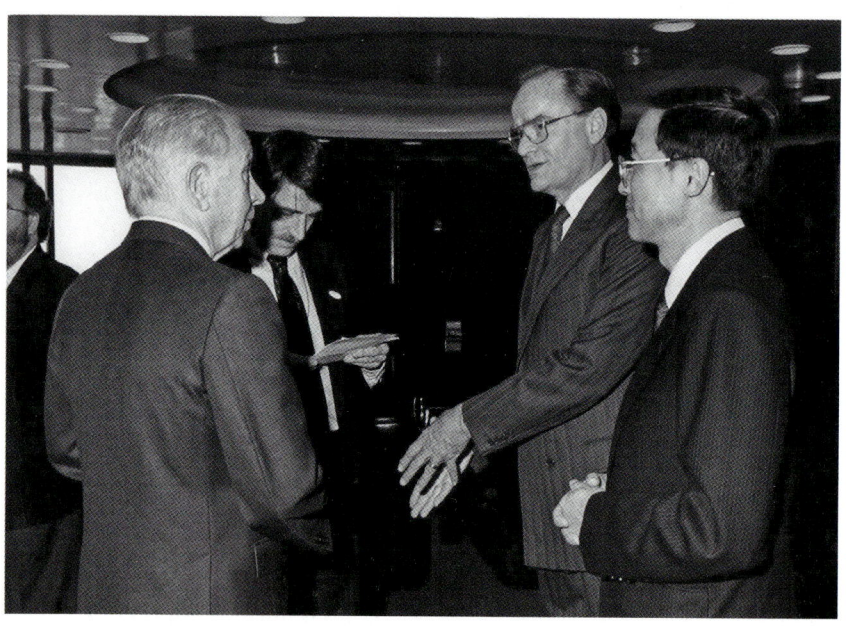

Meeting IOC president Juan Samaranch on home turf in Barcelona in 1995.

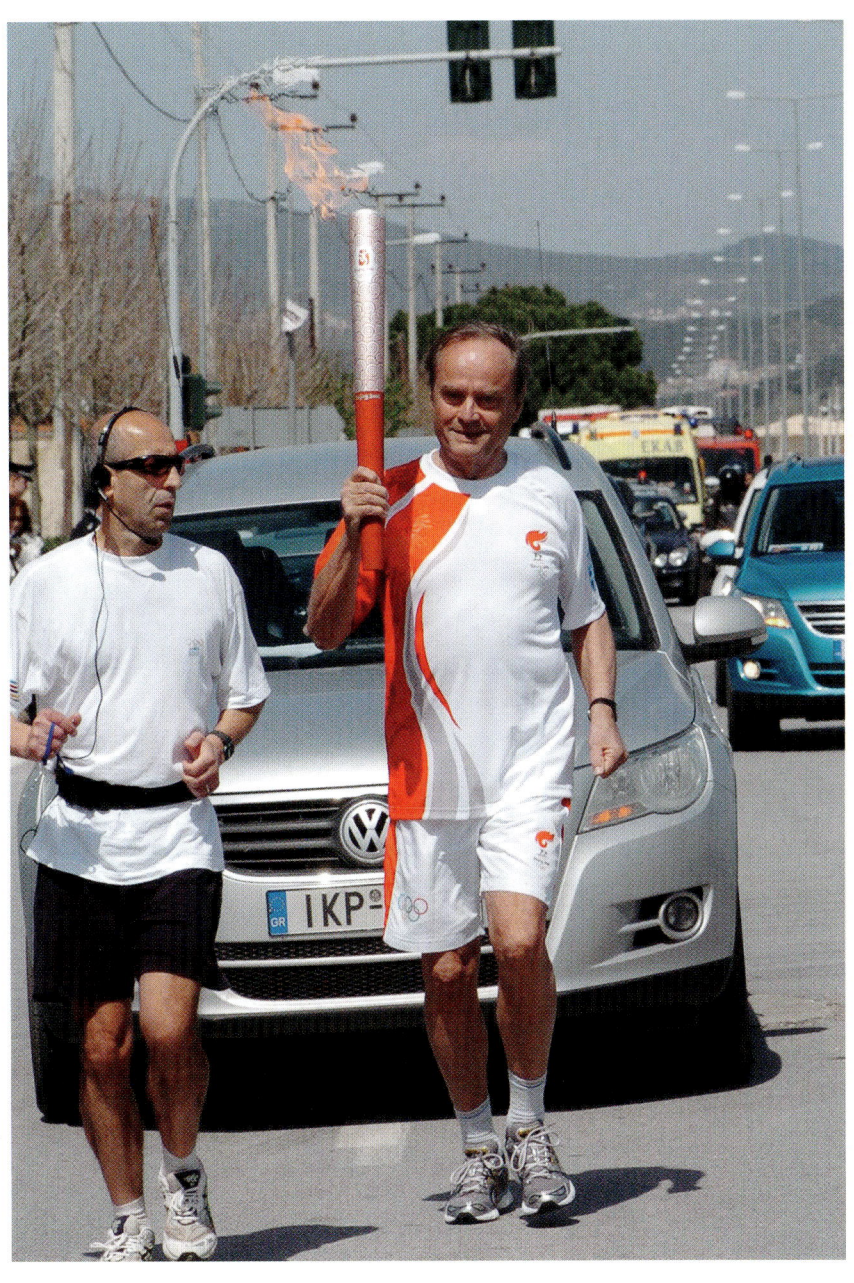

Running through the city of Marathon in 2008 with the olympic flame before it went to China.

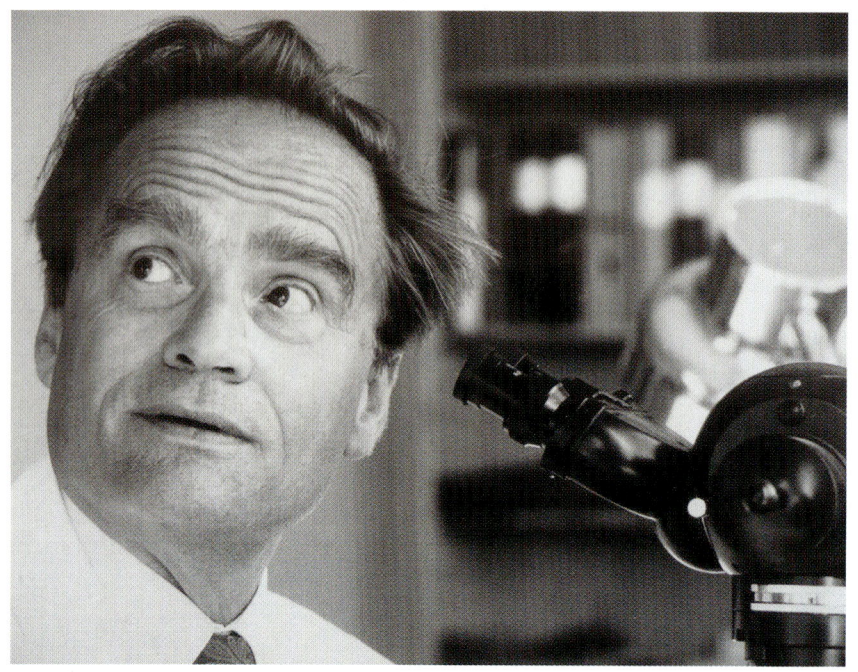

With his professional working instrument, the microscope.

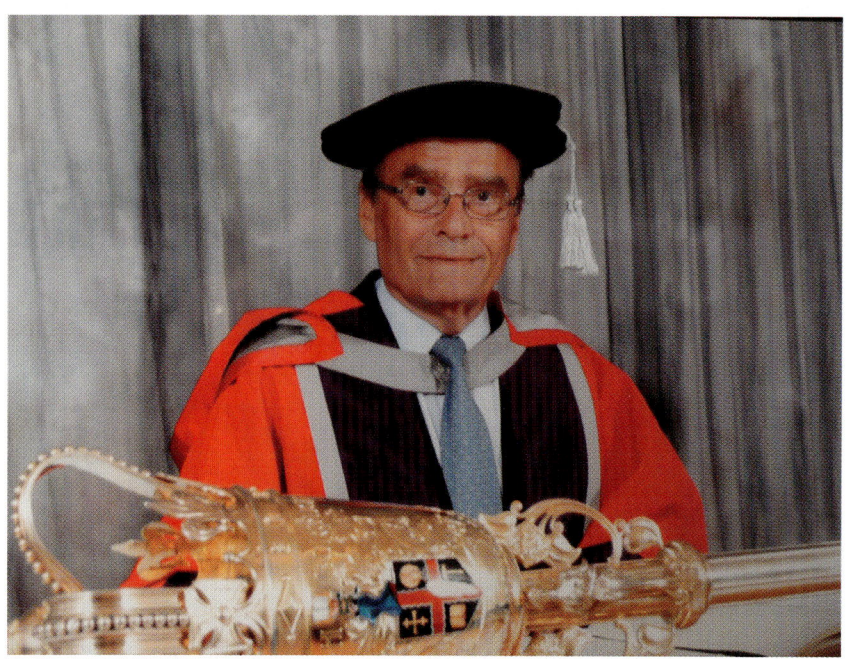

Receiving an Honorary doctorate of Science at the UK's Loughborough University in 2009.

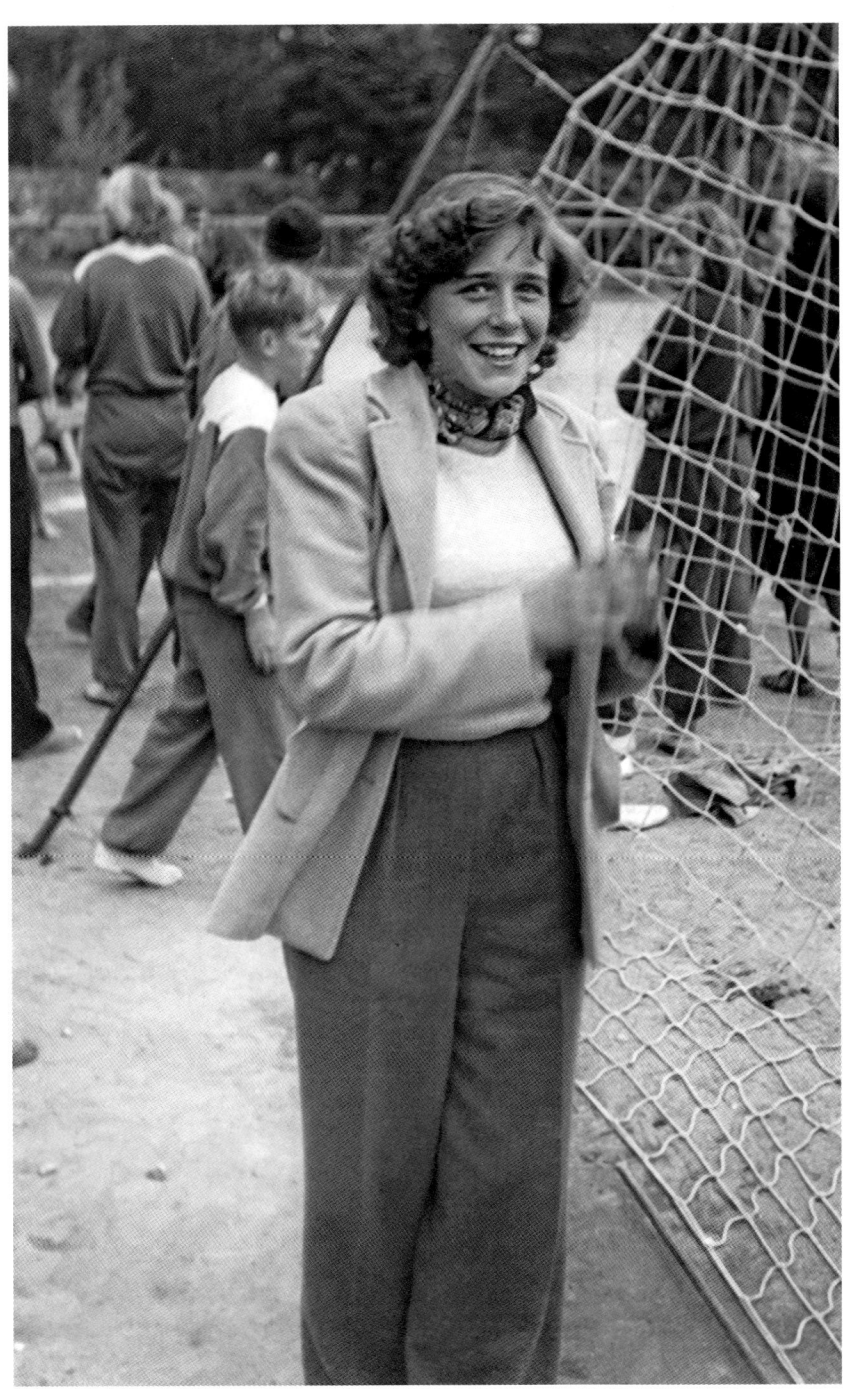

Ulla as a fifteen-year-old spectator at the Stora Mossen sports ground.

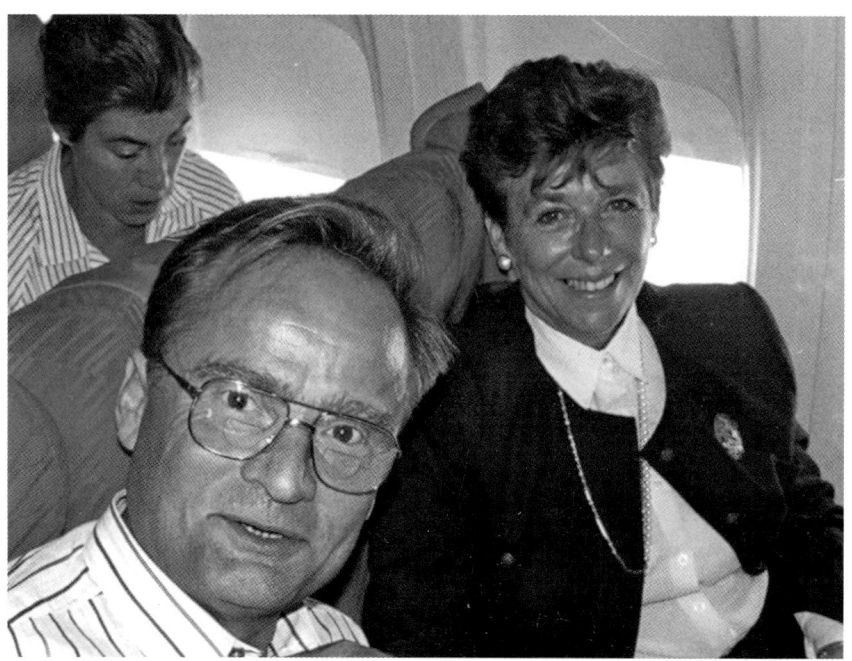

Arne and Ulla travelled around the world. Here in the aeroplane on their way to the IAAF Council meeting in Barcelona in 1989.

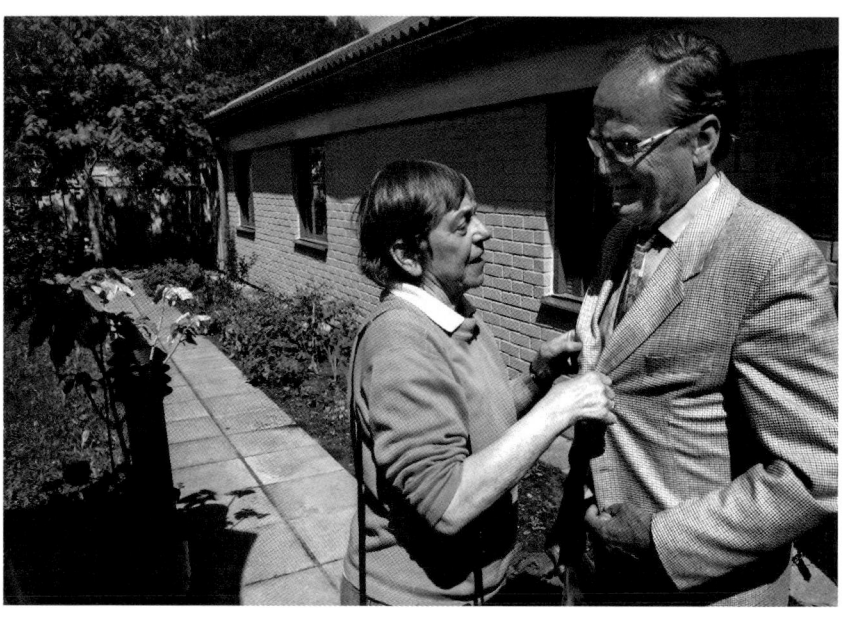

Visiting Ulla in her new living quarters – Smedbygården – in 2006.

doping substances and methods appear. It was impossible to have this kind of long-term planning previously.

'To get an organisation like this up and running is a major undertaking, but it actually went surprisingly smoothly. Key figures at WADA were in place by 2000, and by 2003 a first major task was completed: the common regulations against doping, which is known as the "WADA Code". This came into force at the 2004 Athens Olympics. The IOC demanded that the International Olympic Federations must accept the WADA Code to participate in the Olympic Games.'

WADA is a private foundation, registered in Switzerland. One issue that needed to be resolved quickly was where it should be based. It was agreed that this would be decided by a vote, similar to the way that the Olympic Games host city is chosen. A number of cities applied to have WADA's headquarters.

While the agency was temporarily based in Lausanne, it was not considered the right place for its permanent home because WADA needed to be seen to be separate from the IOC, which also has its headquarters in Lausanne and which, in 2000, was involved in a major corruption scandal.

Early in 2000, two of the leading figures in the Salt Lake City Olympic bid were revealed to have bought votes from members of the IOC, creating the biggest scandal yet for the Olympic movement. Ten IOC members were forced to step down as a result of the accusations.

WADA needed to be distanced from that.

'At the WADA board meeting in Tallinn in 2001, Bonn, Lausanne, Montreal, Stockholm and Vienna applied to be the host city for WADA's head office. I, of course, worked to ensure WADA came to Stockholm. In Sweden, we have a genuine history of working to combat doping, more experience than any other country, in fact. There's considerable knowledge and experience here, not least when it comes to OOC testing.

'Of course, Stockholm also has the Karolinska Institutet, one of the world's leading research centres for biomedicine, somewhere where I have had connections over many years.

'What's more, IDTM also has its headquarters here in Stockholm, so I thought that it would have been a natural move to site WADA's headquarters here.

'Vienna didn't make it because Austria didn't have an accredited laboratory at that time, which was one of the requirements. Then Stockholm, along with Bonn, was ruled out, despite my efforts to convince the panel otherwise. Lausanne was already deemed impossible because of the IOC and the Salt Lake City scandal, but when the European politicians on the board realised that there wasn't any other viable European candidate city left, they then voted for Lausanne.

'Montreal won by a single vote. In April 2002, the WADA headquarters moved to North America.'

DICK POUND, a Canadian lawyer and former Olympic swimmer, was WADA's first president. He was one of the Olympic Movement's leading figures, who had been chairman of the IOC marketing commission for many years. Initially, he was appointed interim WADA president because he was already vice-president of the IOC and was on the IOC executive committee.

'The chairman of the IOC's medical committee, Prince Alexandre de Mérode, was too weak to be the WADA chair. The medical committee's vice-chairman, Jacques Rogge, a Belgian surgeon, was already thought of as likely successor to Samaranch as the IOC president, although Pound was also a candidate. The situation resolved itself when Pound lost the IOC presidency to Rogge, but was offered a new platform at WADA. His legal background was an important asset now that a completely new set of rules and regulations had to be created.'

One of the main tasks for WADA when the agency was created was to put forward an anti-doping code that was acceptable to the IOC, all the international sports federations, and to governments. There were already a number of regulations, so the work didn't need to start from scratch.

The IAAF had a maintained set of rules and regulations that had already been tested in many court cases in different jurisdictions and appeared to be rigorous in that respect. The IOC's own anti-doping code was, however, in many people's eyes a fiasco, full of peculiar things, the result of having been amended in a piecemeal manner too many times.

Richard Young, a legal adviser from the United States Olympic Committee, was appointed to oversee the production of WADA's anti-doping code. Young completed the work in 2003. He based his code to a large extent on the IAAF rules, and Arne was often interviewed and questioned by Young.

In 2003, Young sent his finished, draft code out to more than a hundred anti-doping organisations, national Olympic committees and international sports federations. All of them had the opportunity to give their thoughts on the proposals.

'One of the issues that was most discussed was the different penalties for doping offences. Based on my experience within the IAAF, I wanted penalties that would be legally accepted internationally. Otherwise, we would continue ending up in court around the world.

'That meant that we had to accept that there are different levels of doping offence and that there must also be different penalties. I and the IAAF wanted to have the most severe penalty possible for serious doping offences such as the use of steroids and similar performance-enhancing substances. Other sports federations wanted steroid-use to be penalised on a sliding scale.

'We solved this by reaching a compromise: the most severe penalty to be a two-year ban, with the possibility of reducing it to a one-year ban in exceptional cases. To avoid any loopholes, it was decided that WADA could appeal all penalties.

'A further safety measure which was built into the code was that the board or Executive Committee of WADA were given the power to adjust parts of the code, such as the list of prohibited substances and methods – the banned drugs – which is now reviewed annually.'

The next step was that the governments behind WADA, together with UNESCO (the United Nations Educational, Scientific and Cultrual Organisation), created a convention with the purpose of 'harmonising the global campaign against doping in sport by stressing WADA's mandate as the leading international organisation for combating doping'. The convention would need to be ratified by the United Nations.

'It was not possible to demand that every single country create new laws. Instead, governments decided to tighten this convention within UNESCO. In that way, they pledged to strictly adhere to the contents of the code.'

The convention was finished in October 2005, but for it to come into force it had to be ratified by thirty member states of the UN. It didn't take long to get some countries to sign up, but getting thirty to endorse it took some time.

Sweden was the first country to ratify it, signing within just three weeks. Still, it wasn't until February 1, 2007, that the convention finally came into force, when Luxembourg became the thirtieth country to sign the agreement.

In a press release Lena Adelsohn Liljeroth, Sweden's Minister for Culture, and also responsible for sport, said: 'I am very happy that the UNESCO convention will come into force very soon. The fight against doping within sport is a global fight and demands international co-operation between countries and the sporting movement. It is my belief that all athletes have the right to compete under fair conditions and in a doping-free environment. The UNESCO convention is an important tool to make this possible.'

By October 2010 one hundred and forty eight countries have ratified the convention, representing more than 90 per cent of the world's population.

WADA's CODE CONSISTS of a set of general rules to which are added a series of international standards, among them the list of banned substances and practices. When WADA began its work, a whole host of different lists were in place. Now, they were to be combined to create one uniform list. This work was to be carried out by a committee, responsible for health, medical issues and research within WADA. The chairmanship of the committee was handed to Arne.

'There was no order to the lists at all. New substances had been added to the list, but it hadn't been tidied up nor had anything been taken away. As a result, there were some substances still on the list that could not be considered as a doping substance in any way.

'I can only remember one sole substance that had been taken off the IOC's banned list: that was codeine, which had ended up on the list because in the early days of drug testing it was difficult to distinguish under analysis from morphine. And because codeine was on the list, people assumed that it was a performance-enhancing substance.

'For a substance or practice to end up on the WADA list, it needs to fulfil two out of three criteria: performance-enhancing; dangerous to health; or against the spirit of sport. Therefore, a substance or practice does not need to be performance-enhancing in order to be banned. It is equally important to protect an athlete's health.

'After all, even a regular diet can include some substances that might be viewed to be "performance-enhancing", such as sugar, or different proteins. But when taken in high doses, these harmless foodstuffs can also be dangerous to your health.

'In the end, it comes down to good medical knowledge and commonsense which determines what should or shouldn't be listed. If a case ends up in court, WADA doesn't need to prove that the substance is performance-enhancing, dangerous to health or that it goes against the very nature of sport. Now, the fact that a substance is on the WADA list it regarded as legally binding.

'When the UNESCO convention, connected to the WADA code, came into force we had finally achieved something. Now all the conflict between the world of sport's rules and regulations and national laws was avoidable. It had been a long journey, but in one way it was good to build slowly and surely.'

IN MANY WAYS, the establishment of WADA was the culmination of Arne's journey in sport. When he retired as an athlete from competitive athletics in 1952, no one had heard of doping within Olympic sport. Yet within a decade, the first sporting death directly attributed to drug-use at the Olympic Games occurred when the cyclist Knud Jensen collapsed in Rome in 1960. From then on, the story is one of continuously increasing amounts of doping – a development that was broken only when the IAAF started to act and later when WADA was formed.

'This history is important. There are numerous examples of how much the IOC's rules lacked before the WADA code came into force. At the 1972 Munich Olympic Games, an American swimmer tested positive because he had taken asthma medicine which he was prescribed by his doctor. He was allergic to dust and animal fur.' The swimmer was Rick DeMont and he won the 400 metres freestyle. DeMont was just sixteen years old.

Drug testing in sport was very new in 1972. Then, tests were conducted only at competitions, and then usually only at the biggest events. There were no accepted tests for anabolic steroids, and the banned list at that time comprised almost entirely of stimulants that might be used in competition, of the sort that had contributed to the death of Jensen in 1960.

But as with all drugs on the banned list, the substances usually have an entirely legitimate medical use. In Munich in 1972, the ephedrine that the laboratory found traces of in the urine sample of Rick DeMont was from his prescribed medicine.

In spite of this, the IOC decided to strip DeMont of his gold medal. The outcome perhaps would have been different if DeMont, or his team officials, had notified IOC that the swimmer needed to take ephedrine and they had had it approved by the IOC's medical committee beforehand. But in those early days of drug testing, the people around DeMont hadn't thought about it, maybe because there weren't any clear rules.

'This was before my time. My first Olympics as an international sports official was 1976, when I took up my post at the IAAF. On that occasion it was a runner and seven weightlifters who failed their drug tests with traces of anabolic steroids. Thankfully, that was more clear-cut than what had happened to Rick DeMont during the Munich Games.

'But then four years later still, at the 1980 Moscow Olympics, there wasn't a single positive drug test at all. Moscow was a completely "clean" Olympics.

'Of course, the United States boycotted those Games, along with sixty-four other nations from the West in protest against the Soviet Union's invasion of Afghanistan. But the Moscow Games were not quite so "clean".

'After the Olympics, Professor Manfred Donike, from the testing laboratory in Cologne, did his own, additional analyses on the urine samples collected in Moscow. These unofficial tests suggested that the 1980 Games were far from "clean".

'When I went to the 1984 Los Angeles Olympics, it was in the dual capacity of vice-president of the IAAF and chairman of the medical committee. There, I witnessed something that was startling, but when I later responded, I was bawled out by Primo Nebiolo.'

In Los Angeles, the Finns had shown their strength in the long-distance races through Martti Vainio, who came second in the 10,000 metres. He was also a good 5000 metres runner who had won the bronze medal at the first IAAF world championships, staged in Helsinki the previous year, and so was among the favourites to win the gold in Los Angeles.

As one of the medal-winners in the 10,000 metres final, Vainio had to give a urine sample for analysis. Before that sample had been analysed at the laboratory, Vainio had raced again in the 5000 metres heats and qualified for the final.

But on the morning of that final, the head of the Finnish delegation, Carl-Olaf Homen, telephoned Arne. Homen told Arne that Vainio had tested positive for steroids. Arne advised him that Vainio should be excluded from the 5000 metres. But Vainio refused to withdraw.

'I had to act on my own. I went to Fred Holder, who was the IAAF's technical delegate and in charge of the competition as far as the IAAF was concerned. Just before the 5000 metres final, together with Carl-Olaf Homen, we walked over to the warm-up area and took Vainio off the track. It wasn't clear if we could do this, on the basis of just one A sample test, before the secondary, B sample had been analysed.'

It has long been the practice in doping control that when collecting a sample from a competitor for testing, the urine provided is immediately split in to two separate containers, 'A' and 'B', with the competitor witnessing this happening. Both bottles are sent securely, and anonymously, to the laboratory, where the first portion of the sample is analysed. If this proves negative for any traces of banned drugs, the athlete has no case to answer and no further action is taken. The second portion of the urine sample, the 'B sample', is then not required.

However, if there is what is called an 'adverse finding' by the lab in the analysis of the first, 'A sample', then as a legal safety check, the athlete, their team management and advisers, may attend the laboratory to witness the analysis of this secondary 'B sample' to ensure that all proper procedures are followed and that the outcome of the second analysis matches the first.

Back in Los Angeles in 1984, Vainio's 5000 metres final was about to be held before it had been possible to arrange for the runner and the Finnish team officials to attend the lab to witness this secondary part of the procedure.

'There weren't any clear rules at that time, but I acted as I thought best. That evening, I was at a garden party that Primo Nebiolo also attended. He came over to me and gently took me to one side, for a private conversation, I thought.

'But what followed was far from a conversation.

'He gave me a real ticking off for acting on my initiative. I defended my actions, though: it could have been much worse if it had got out that the IAAF knew that the Finn had tested positive and yet still let him compete in an Olympic final. For a long time Vainio denied that he had ever doped, but finally had to admit that he had actually done so.

'I never really believed that doping was particularly important on Nebiolo's agenda. At least not at that time. He was more concerned about what the world thought of the IAAF. Having overall leadership of athletics and sport's independence was what he really ached for.

'But four years later, he gave me his full support to act independently during the Ben Johnson scandal. And it was Primo who persuaded Samaranch that I should become a member of the IOC's medical committee in 1987.

'So it was thanks to Primo that I was there in 1988 when the Winter Olympics took place in Calgary. And it was on the eve of those Games that I first spoke to Samaranch about the idea of creating a foundation to finance research in the field of anti-doping.'

There was an ongoing discussion within the IOC medical committee about new forms of doping and medication. The need to develop methods of analysis for the new medication that were continually appearing on the black market was constant. Expensive research was needed to do this.

At the end of the 1980s, it was blood doping using erythropoietin, or EPO, which was the next big threat to sport.

Erythropoietin is a naturally occurring human hormone which normally stimulates the production of red blood cells. It is the volume of these cells which determine the body's capacity for carrying oxygen to the muscles: with more red blood cells, the blood stream can carry more oxygen to the muscles, a vital element for athletes competing in endurance events, such as distance running, swimming, cycling and cross-country skiing.

'We sat there in 1988 discussing the risk that EPO might be available as a doping agent, long before we had any way of identifying that the substance had been administered artificially to help sportsmen cheat. As things turned out, it would take eleven years before we found a reliable test to uncover EPO doping. It would have happened much sooner if we had been able to initiate and support research.

'In my eyes, it was almost scandalous that the IOC didn't provide research funds much earlier. When I talked to Samaranch on the eve of Calgary in 1988, he told me that he thought my suggestion was excellent, but that there was an established formula for the distribution of the money which the IOC made from television and sponsorship of the Olympics, which people would not like to change. Nebiolo thought the same.

'In fact, everyone thought it was a great idea, but no one wanted to give up any part of their share of the Olympic TV money. It was only when WADA was founded that funds were finally allocated for research out of the agency's own budget.'

The thing was, by then, Olympic sport, including athletics, had already been rocked by some of the biggest doping scandals in history.

Chapter 10

Ben Johnson, Sotomayor and the Rest

THE CALGARY WINTER Olympics was a kind of a warm up for Arne, to ready him for the responsibilities of overseeing the drug-testing system ahead of the summer Games that would take place later the same year in Seoul, South Korea. There, Arne was to carry the main responsibility for doping controls in athletics, in what was to become one of the greatest scandals in sporting history.

It was during the Seoul Games that Ben Johnson would beat Carl Lewis in the blue riband of the track, the 100 metres. The American, dubbed 'King Carl' in the press, had won four gold medals in Los Angeles and came to Seoul determined to defend his titles.

The year before, in Rome, at the IAAF world championships, Johnson, of Canada, had beaten Lewis in the 100 metres final, running 9.83 seconds to set a world record. Lewis was stunned by the defeat and immediately after the race he made allegations about drug-use in a television interview, although carefully he named no names.

The rivalry between the Canadian and American bubbled away all through the European track season of 1988, with Lewis ultimately coming out on top when the two men clashed in Zurich, the last important meeting before the Olympics. 'The gold medal for the 100 metres is mine,' said Lewis, looking ahead to the Olympics. 'I will never again lose to Johnson.'

In the Olympic 100 metres final in Seoul, Lewis finished one and a half metres behind Johnson, as the Canadian smashed his own world record, running 9.79 seconds.

But Johnson was doped.

The revelations that would come out during and after those Seoul Olympics shocked the entire world of sport. 'I think that the Johnson scandal became a turning point in the work against doping. It was like an alarm clock that woke everyone up.'

ARNE HAD FIRST met Lewis at the start of his career, and he recognised that he would become a great role model and because of that a great help in the fight against doping.

'It was 1981 at the World Cup in Rome. In the stadium I sat next to Ollan Cassell, the then chief executive of USA Track and Field, who was a close friend of mine. He told me about an eighteen-year-old who was going to compete who he said was going to be a big world star.

'It was Carl Lewis. I remember well that he competed in the long jump in Rome. I met him two years later at the world championships in Helsinki and made sure I took him to one side to talk to him.

'When we were on our own I told him about the extent to which athletics and sport were under threat from drugs and doping. I told him I thought he could help in the fight against doping and that he could be an excellent role model.

'I thought that it would be wonderful to get a young man like this on our side. I don't know if Lewis remembers everything I said on that occasion, but his coach did. Joe Douglas came up to me and reminded me of that day in 1983 on several occasions. After that, Lewis was a committed supporter of the anti-doping programme.

'Because of that, I was dismayed to pick up a Norwegian newspaper after the 1983 world championships and see the headline: "Carl Lewis doped at Helsinki world championships".

'I should have been the first to know something like this, but I hadn't heard a thing. It was an unfounded rumour. It's dreadful the kind of damage that sort of journalism does when they throw all sorts of unfounded suspicions around. There are always stacks of people that swallow these headlines hook, line and sinker, believing them.

'I can't say that I know Carl Lewis. In fact, it's very difficult to get to know him. But I've followed his career since Rome in 1981, and still follow him. The last time that I met him was at the IAAF Gala in Monte Carlo in 2007.

'In my eyes he is one of the greatest athletes of all time. Ten Olympic medals, nine gold and one silver. And eleven world championship medals: eight gold, two silver and one bronze. He was crowned sportsman of the year in 1983, 1984, and 1991. Carl Lewis can be compared to Jesse Owens. But look what happened to him: he was outrun by a man who cheated.'

BEN JOHNSON'S ABBREVIATED career caught people's attention a long time before the Seoul Olympics. Rumours that he was doping abounded, but at that time the only thing that could prove if an athlete was doped or not was a positive drugs test. Without such evidence, there was nothing that anyone in authority could say.

'Ahead of the competitions I met Ben Johnson at a reception for those competing, and when I saw his eyes, I was a bit uneasy. The whites of his eye were very yellow, a sign that the rumours were true. Steroids taken orally affect the liver when used over a long period of time.'

Of all the events in the Olympic Games, the 100 metres final is the most spectacular. Although Johnson had broken the world record in Rome a year earlier, Lewis was still favourite to win when they met in Seoul.

For the final, Arne sat in the main stand of Seoul's Olympic Stadium and was able to follow from close range. There, he saw that Lewis did not stand a chance as Johnson broke his own world record.

'I hurried down straight after the final to the doping control station where the drug tests took place. It was the Seoul organising committee that carried out the actual tests, but I was there to advise them and ensure that everything followed protocol.

'So there I sat, waiting for Ben Johnson and his accompanying persons to come. And when he finally got there he had a hoard of people with him.

'I've never seen such a circus. With the help of one of the Koreans, we managed to get rid of his screeching hangers-on. Then we remained sitting face-to-face: Johnson, his physiotherapist, and I. We just sat there staring at each other until Johnson was ready to go into the small room to give his urine sample. He went in and did it and then left the premises. An analysis takes one day. When I returned to the hotel the next evening with Ulla, there was an envelope under the door. I opened it and read. Ben Johnson's A test was positive. Traces of the anabolic steroid Stanozolol had been found.

'Ulla asked what it was. "Nothing special," I told her. It's essential to keep everything regarding a test result confidential. The only other people notified about the test result were the big cheeses within the IAAF and IOC. But when the Canadian Olympic Committee was informed sometime after midnight, complete panic broke out.'

The following day, Johnson's B sample was analysed. It confirmed that Johnson had taken Stanozolol. He was to be questioned that evening by the medical committee at the IOC's official hotel, the Shilla. After that, the medical committee would give their recommendation to the IOC's executive board about what measures were to be taken.

One of those who hurried to Johnson's defence was Dick Pound. At that time, Pound was a member of the IOC's executive board, but he also represented the Canadian Olympic Committee. He was also a very successful lawyer.

Pound led the Canadian delegation. His argument was that the test had been interfered with and that this could have happened because the security at the doping station had completely fallen apart.

'I was almost new on the medical committee when I was confronted by Pound, but I was well-prepared. Earlier in the day, I had talked to the Professor Arnold Beckett, the medical committee member from Britain. He had also heard the rumour that the defence was going to focus on the chaos when Johnson arrived at the doping control station.

'So I asked Pound which security had been breached. He answered that people had come into the waiting room who shouldn't have been there. I replied that at no point do the IOC rules and regulations stipulate who should be or who shouldn't be allowed in the doping control station's waiting room; it only states who is allowed to be in the room where the sample is taken. I also informed him that Johnson had been in view the entire time.

Pound's attempt to discredit us lacked weight, and when Manfred Donike said that Johnson's urine sample revealed long-term use of Stanozolol, the defence didn't have a leg to stand on. Pound understood this.

'We bumped into each other again the next day and he made a point of thanking me for the day before and that we had sorted things out.

'At the Olympics, world championships, and similar events, rumours and allegations of doping often circulate. I don't know how many times I've had to put such rumours to bed. It's not so easy because I'm really not allowed to say anything as long as a particular case is under investigation. But if I don't dispel a rumour, it is taken as an indication that it's true.

'In Seoul there were rumours circulating that Johnson was doped. Had someone seen the Canadian delegation come to the Hotel Shilla that evening? Or had there been a leak? Later, we learned that there was a leak. Late at night, before the IOC went public, I was woken by knocking at the door of my hotel room. There was a Swedish journalist outside wanting a comment about the rumours. I asked the journalist to leave as I needed to sleep, and I closed the door on him. I think it's the only time I've been explicitly unfriendly to a journalist. How on earth he got past the hotel security is still a mystery to me.'

The IOC's executive board decided that Johnson should be stripped of his medal, disqualified and sent home. After that it was a matter for the IAAF and Athletics Canada – the national federation – to decide how long Ben Johnson should be banned from athletics. 'The ball was first in the IAAF's court and they organised a press conference which Nebiolo would hold the same day as the IOC went public with the news that Ben Johnson had tested positive for doping and was being disqualified from the Olympics. The press conference took place at the IAAF hotel.

'Nebiolo asked me to accompany him in his car from the Shilla to the IAAF hotel. On the way to the press conference something unexpected happened. Nebiolo usually loved to appear in front of the cameras, but now he said to me: "You can take this press conference, Arne."

'He clearly realised that he would have trouble explaining exactly what had happened and that he was going to be faced with some tough questions. When we arrived at the hotel it turned out that the press conference had needed to be moved from the intended conference room to the large hotel lobby because there were so many journalists present. Standing on a makeshift podium in front of the world's press and a forest of microphones worthy of an American presidential appearance, I had to explain what had happened and what would follow. In the audience, Nebiolo sat listening.

'It was nerve-racking, of course, but it went well. It was my first, big international press conference, a baptism of fire that I would be able to draw on during the many similar situations I would find myself in later on.'

The Ben Johnson scandal was a national catastrophe for Canada. The Canadian government, which had always invested generously in the country's Olympic sportsmen and women, decided to stage a judicial inquiry to ascertain what had happened and, importantly, to learn how something similar could be avoided in the future.

The inquiry took the form of a kind of court trial, with far reaching authority. There would be a prosecuting attorney, and the witnesses were called to testify under oath. They were entitled to have legal representation with them. Charles Dubin, the Ontario Appeal Court Chief Justice, was appointed as judge and it was he who led the inquiry. Robert Armstrong, a senior lawyer and Queen's Counsel, was appointed as prosecutor.

Among the many witnesses, Arne was called to the trial in Toronto and was assisted there by a Canadian lawyer. 'It was Armstrong himself who called me in the spring of 1989 and told me that the hearing would take place at some point in September. When I was actually sitting there in the courtroom, it was apparent that Armstrong's tactic was to accuse the IAAF and IOC of not taking a firm enough grip on the question of doping. We had apparently ignored the problem and under the prevalent circumstances, Johnson was left with no other choice but to use banned substances.

'I pointed out that their argument was deeply unfair and full of insinuations. I gave an account of the IAAF's already then ambitious anti-doing programme. But I had to work really hard to dispel all the accusations. Johnson's coach Charlie Francis admitted that he well remembered taking care of Johnson's doping programme for almost nine years, although Johnson himself continually maintained in Seoul that he had never knowingly taken any banned substance. Johnson maintained this at the first press conference after the IOC's decision in Seoul and continued to do so whenever asked thereafter.'

Johnson was banned for two years. Because of the admissions of long-term doping that he and Charlie Francis made under oath to the Dubin Inquiry, he was stripped not only of his Olympic title and the world record set in the race in Seoul, after which he tested positive, but also stripped of his 1987 world title, and his world record performance in that race was also erased.

It was the first time that any retrospective sanction had been applied as a consequence of someone's admission of doping.

When Johnson's ban ended in 1991, he attempted to make a comeback. He was subjected to regular drug tests, in and out of competition, and eventually he again tested positive, this time for testosterone. 'We arranged a press conference again, this time in Paris. We were met by the same scepticism once more, the same attempts to discredit the tests, the same claim that it was not possible to establish conclusively that it was testosterone. The IAAF, however, saw this as a clear cut case of doping. The positive test was the only proof that was needed. It was left to Athletics Canada to penalise him.'

As was expected for any second offence, Johnson was handed a life ban.

'I know that he did some running against horses and suchlike in some kind of circus. It's tragic and pathetic.'

'BEN JOHNSON WAS the wake-up call. I can compare it to how it was in Sweden before and after Linda Haglund. Before Linda tested positive, I'm not sure anyone cared about doping, but as soon as there was a ruling in that case, opinion changed. Having first protected her and criticised us, people started to understand what we were doing.

'After the Johnson scandal, the entire world's opinion changed about doping in sport.'

It is even possible to see that the Johnson case helped make WADA a reality. But it took more than a decade, and during the 1990s, the inadequate rules and regulations of the IOC, IAAF and others continued to cause problems.

Just in time for the 1992 Barcelona Olympics, Clenbuterol emerged as a popular doping substance. It is a substance that is not classified as a steroid, but it has a similar effect. Ahead of the Games, several athletes had tested positive for the substance, including two British weightlifters. When this became known, one of the members of the IOC's medical committee, Professor Arnold Beckett, from London, stated publicly that Clenbuterol should not be banned.

This was after the East German sprinters Katrin Krabbe and Grit Breuer had tested positive for that very substance and been forced to drop out. 'Beckett's reaction was upsetting, of course. You could say that he disqualified himself. Prince de Mérode, the chairman of the IOC's medical committee, was furious and fired Beckett from the committee even though he was a world-leading figure within the anti-doping movement and the holder of an honorary doctorate from Uppsala University, and so on. Naturally, the doped British weightlifters were not allowed to compete at the Olympics.'

But there were new doping substances appearing all the time. It was only when WADA began to support research that there was at least a chance to keep up with the dopers. Until then it was necessary to combat the new substances with new and unproved methods of analysis.

'We were faced with an example of this kind of problem leading up to the 1996 Olympic Games in Atlanta. A new method of analysis had been developed called HRMS – High Resolution Mass Spectrometry. With the help of this, it was possible to trace minute levels of steroids much more accurately than with the old mass spectrometry.'

The method had been developed for the purpose of doping analysis by Professor Manfred Donike, at the IOC-accredited laboratory in Cologne. Donike had always been at the forefront when it came to research and development.

Before the Olympics in 1996, samples from weightlifters were analysed in Cologne with the HRMS-method. The analysis revealed itself to be effective: several weightlifters were caught with steroids in their bodies.

'After that, the International Weightlifting Federation (IWF) wanted HRMS testing to be made a prerequisite technique for doping labs to be accredited. It was completely unrealistic. It takes a long time to refine and test new methods of analysis.

'But Samaranch came under strong pressure from the IWF; they had had such "positive" experiences with HRMS that they considered that all tests should be done with it in Atlanta. Samaranch called me in the spring of 1996 and asked my opinion. I replied that a laboratory required a longer running-in period before it could handle a whole Olympics with a new technique.

'In spite of this, it was decided that the Atlanta lab should use HRMS. I don't know why. Perhaps the decision was taken after even more pressure being applied by the IWF.'

It was not until after the Atlanta Games that Arne noticed that some strange things were happening over the drug testing at the Olympics. 'We had gone home and were waiting for the test results from the last few days of the Games, but they never arrived.

'I wrote to Prince de Mérode, enquiring about the final reports, but again received no answer. After a while, the head of the Atlanta laboratory, Don Catlin, made a statement to the press appealing for the final test results to be released. He knew that there were three or four samples that were positive.

'The question was taken up within the IAAF. Naturally, we were concerned that the positive results may have come from our athletes, given that the final days of the Olympic Games are a culmination of the athletics events. Obviously, people asked me questions about it, but I could only reply that I knew nothing. This in turn, of course, surprised and concerned my friends on the IAAF Council.'

The only thing Arne could show was that he had written to Prince de Mérode, but not received an answer despite reminding him. When the story at last leaked to the press there was, of course, considerable coverage. There was a new air of scandal. When the press coverage reached Samaranch he, in turn, wrote a letter to Arne asking why he had criticised his own committee chairman. 'It was an illustration of how afraid of conflict he was. The Olympic family had to appear together at least outwardly. "Of course.' I thought to myself, "but not at any price."'

Finally, the truth came out. The final tests really had been positive, but they had been tested using the HRMS method. Prince de Mérode, who was still in Atlanta after the Games, had along with some medical commission members, decided to declare the results invalid as the method of testing was new and not properly validated before Atlanta.

'A NEW SUBSTANCE turned up in our tests in Atlanta. We had been aware of it already ahead of the Olympic Games. Bromantan was a stimulant used by the Russian military, but it wasn't on our banned list even though it was classified as a stimulant and was clearly taken with a view to doping. The medical committee recommended that the Russian athletes caught using Bromantan should be banned.

'They were banned by the IOC executive board but the ruling was subject to an appeal at the highest level, the Court for Arbitration in Sport, or CAS. Unbelievably, CAS completely exonerated them. So now the IOC's medical committee had to hurry up with getting Bromantan on the list of banned substances.'

The Atlanta Olympics revealed several weaknesses in the legal procedures for dealing with doping cases, as demonstrated by Italian high jumper Antonella Bevilacqua who, in the May before the Olympics, tested positive for pseudoephedrine and ephedrine and yet was exonerated by the Italian national athletics federation. The IAAF could have argued that the Italians' ruling was incorrect and taken the case to its arbitration panel, but because the panel didn't convene before the Olympic Games, she was allowed to compete.

'It was dreadful. A jumper who had unequivocally tested positive was allowed to compete in an Olympic event. What's more, she was a favourite for a medal.

'Supported by Nebiolo, I tried to convince the chairman of the Italian federation that she should not compete, but he refused to listen. It was on the verge of putting me in a highly precarious position. I was to present the medals in the women's high jump, and there was a risk I would be handing one to a high jumper who rightly shouldn't receive it.

'I was saved on the goal line by a completely unknown jumper from Greece who had the event of her life and, setting a personal record of 2.03 metres, snatched the silver medal, knocking Bevilacqua into fourth.

'But I still didn't award the medals. Immediately after the final, the Greek IOC member Nikos Filaretos, came over to me and asked if he could replace me as the prize-giver in the high jump. Of course he could, and he became my friend for life.'

Bevilacqua was banned for three months when her case was eventually taken up by the arbitration panel, following which the official Olympic results were amended and her name deleted from the record.

'But we couldn't have things like this happening. We couldn't have an arbitration panel that didn't convene when we needed it, and allow things like the Bevilacqua case to occur. We decided then that the panel would be on hand, ready to convene at every major event like a world championships or Olympic Games.

'In Sydney in 2000, the same thing happened as in Atlanta. A new kind of analysis was developed, this time to expose doping with erythropoietin, EPO, but we hadn't come far enough in validating it for the analytical approach to be scientifically and legally valid. It was the Paris lab that had developed a new way of spotting the recent use of EPO. It was based on Swedish research findings that had been carried out by a professor of chemistry at Uppsala University, Leif Wide, the son of the former running champion and Olympic medallist in the 1920s, Edvin Wide.

'A research group in Sydney had, at the same time, discovered an alternative method that could ascertain whether an athlete was doped with EPO by measuring their blood count.

'In order for an analysis method to be validated it needs to be peer reviewed and published in an international scientific journal and then confirmed by researchers independent of the initial study, who in turn publish their own findings. It is a sometimes long and complicated process, but necessary.

'The Australians wanted us to speed up the validation process of blood analysis, so we put together an expert group in the summer of 2000. They agreed that the analysis results from urine tests were scientifically acceptable if the tests could be "supported" by clear signs of an abnormally high blood count. In other words, we needed a combination of the methods developed in Paris and Sydney.'

At that time, drug testing had only ever been done by using urine testing, regarded as a 'non-invasive' method.

Taking blood samples, an 'invasive' method, was another complicated area of human rights law.

'In the end, the methods did not work satisfactorily at the Sydney Games. But we made use of the experience at the Winter Olympics in Salt Lake City two years later. And that was really lucky: everyone in Sweden remembers long-distance skier Johan Muehlegg, who beat the Swedes to medals but was then disqualified. He was caught using a completely new variant of EPO.'

German-born Muehlegg, skiing for Spain, had been called in for a doping test straight after his gold-winning 50-kilometres race, but the urine sample he gave could not be used for testing as it was too dilute. On his way to the doping control station after his event, Muehlegg had urinated and then had drunk lots of water.

'Naturally, we became suspicious. But we decided to let him think that the test was okay. We nabbed him again, later that evening at the medal ceremony, and then he didn't have a spare minute to go and pee. That test contained traces of NESP, a new, artificial variant of EPO.

'It was right in the middle of the Games when Don Catlin, the head of the testing laboratory, asked me to come over to the lab: he had something to show me. He had found NESP in one of the samples.'

Within the anti-doping regulations, the term 'related substance' is used as a fall-back just in case there hasn't been time to update the list of banned substances. Thanks to this rule, NESP could be taken as a 'related substance' to EPO. Muehlegg left the Olympics accompanied by two female cross-country skiers from Russia who also tested positive for NESP. NESP had only been around for a couple of months but cheats could still be banned for using it. It was one of the first signs that the doping hunters were hot on the heels of the cheats.

AT THE 2000 Sydney Olympics, the Cuban high jumper Javier Sotomayor competed, despite testing positive for cocaine at the Pan American Games in Winnipeg the previous year. He had been banned for two years. 'But ahead of the Sydney Olympic Games a request was received that his ban should be reduced as he had "done so much for world athletics".

'Amazingly enough, the majority of my colleagues on the council of the IAAF accepted his appeal and reduced the ban. I was very close to leaving my post at the IAAF in protest against the decision.

'It was Professor Eduardo de Rose from the Pan American medical committee who was responsible for the tests in Winnipeg who then went on to ensure that Sotomayor was disqualified from the Pan American Games. The IAAF then, in accordance with the rules, forwarded the matter to the Cuban federation to decide whether he should be banned for two years, but the case prompted considerable protests.'

Sotomayor was national hero in Cuba, having twice won the world title and also gold at the Barcelona Olympics, as well as setting the world record 2.45 metres in 1993, a mark which still stood in 2011. As such, Sotomayor was a favourite of Cuba's President, Fidel Castro, who dismissed the positive drug test as a CIA-inspired Western conspiracy to discredit a great Cuban.

'The decision in Winnipeg was labelled "political", although this wasn't the case. People were talking about sabotage, but we had evidence to show that that wasn't so. Fidel Castro even gave a speech on TV addressing the nation, defending Sotomayor. Cuba's representative at the IAAF, Alberto Juantorena, the legendary runner who went on to become Cuba's Minister of Sport, made a considerable point of defending his countryman.

'In spite of this Sotomayor was, nonetheless, banned for two years.'

It wasn't the first time that this problem had been faced. The doping laboratory had a positive test, which ought to be the end of the matter. It is the only evidence that is required. But suddenly the board of the IAAF convened and gave Juantorena their support and reduced Sotomayor's ban. 'I made a strong reservation against this decision, of course, and much later I had the opportunity to talk about the incident with the new IAAF president, Lamine Diack. He admitted that he hadn't been in possession of all the facts when the decision was taken and so, with hindsight, admitted that he and the Council had been wrong and that I was right.'

So there was Javier Sotomayor at the high jump in Sydney, convicted of doping and he hadn't even served the ban he was given. This was sneered upon by the public and fellow athletes. The lanky, tall world record-holder, had pushed Sweden's Patrik Sjöberg into second place in the all-time rankings.

'To let him compete was like a slap in the face for everyone who fought for drug-free athletics, a slap in the face for everyone who competed in the same Olympic event.

'Sotomayor won the silver medal in Sydney, knocking the Swedish athlete Stefan Holm into fourth place. Naturally, Holm was justifiably bitter about missing out on an Olympic medal because the IAAF had reduced Sotomayor's ban.'

In 2001, Sotomayor tested positive again. This time, it was for the anabolic steroid nandrolone. This was the end of the road for him as a high jumper. And Holm got his Olympic redemption when he won the gold medal at the Athens Games in 2004.

Chapter 11

The Big Battle

ONE OF THE biggest obstacles in combating the use of drugs in sport is people's national loyalty. The history of anti-doping is littered with examples of how national federations with misguided loyalties have got behind their own people when they have been caught blatantly doping. They forget that it is their responsibility to protect all the athletes who are not doping.

Almost without exception when these instances occur, 'procedural errors' are blamed. This leads to drawn-out and expensive legal processes, often with absurd consequences. Sport's international federations are often sidelined, watching as the national governing body tries to run the disciplinary process.

'Briefly, this is what happens. A doping test is usually a urine sample that is divided into two bottles: an A sample and a B sample. They are sent by secure, registered courier to a WADA-approved laboratory. The lab does not know who the samples are from – if the tests have been conducted by WADA or the IOC, or the national anti-doping agency, the lab will not even know what sport is involved.

'Once the A portion of the urine sample is analysed, the result is sent to whoever has ordered the test and, nowadays, a copy of the results are even sent to WADA as well as the relevant international sports federation. If the analysis is positive, then further administrative checks are undertaken to ascertain if the athlete has a "Therapeutic Use Exemption", what we call a TUE, for the banned substance that has been detected.

'If no TUE exists, then the athlete is advised of the adverse finding and given an opportunity to explain him or herself. If the explanation is not acceptable, the athlete is adjudged to be doped, but has the right to have the B sample analysed in his or her presence. If the analysis of the B sample does not confirm the findings of the A test, then the case is dismissed.

'But if the B test confirms the findings of the A test, then the national federation whose jurisdiction the competitor is under is supposed to hand out a penalty in accordance with the applicable regulations. It is often at this point that the problems begin ...

'While the national federations pledge their loyalty to the work being done to tackle doping in sport, they might claim that in this instance, something has gone wrong or that there are special circumstances to take into consideration and that the competitor should be handed a milder punishment than stipulated in the rules. Often they argue that their competitor should be cleared completely.

'If the international federation finds that the penalty imposed by the national federation on its athlete is not in-keeping with the regulations, then it can rule on the correct penalty (this applies to some international federations) or it can pass the case on to CAS (which applies, for example, to the IAAF). Even WADA can appeal to CAS.'

One of the national governing bodies which was notorious for protecting its own athletes, even if they were doped, was the Americans, known today as USA Track & Field (USATF). Up until 1992, it was called The Athletics Congress (TAC).

A blatant example was the case of Mary Decker-Slaney, one of the world's foremost middle-distance runners.

She was America's darling from the time that, as a precocious fourteen-year-old dubbed 'Little Mary Decker', she famously battled to a 800 metres victory in a 1973 'dual meet' against the Soviet Union. As she got older, her career suffered several set-backs, both through injury and the 1980 American-led boycott of the Moscow Olympic Games. Undaunted, between 1980 and 1982 she still managed to break world records at three distances, the mile, 5,000 and 10,000 metres, and in 1984 she arrived at the Olympics in Los Angeles in 1984 having won the gold in both the 1,500 and 3,000 metres at the 1983 world championships.

The American dream was for Mary Slaney – by then married to a British discus thrower, Richard Slaney – to win the Olympic gold for the 3,000 metres. But in the final, Slaney tripped over Zola Budd, the South African-born barefooted runner competing for Britain, leaving the darling of all America weeping on the side of the track. An entire nation cried with her, it seemed.

Twelve years later, she got another shot at winning an Olympic medal on her home soil, in Atlanta. But by now thirty-seven, she was apparently past her best and did not even make the final of the 5000 metres.

Yet Slaney carried on competing, and in Paris the following spring, at the IAAF World Indoor Championships, she finished second in the 1,500 metres final to win the silver medal. Then it was revealed that she had been doped.

The year before, Slaney had produced an adverse testosterone test at the US Olympic trials *before* the Atlanta Games, but USATF decided not to take any action. Slaney could have been banned for two years, but the Americans let her continue competing as if nothing had happened.

'It was in the midst of a generation shift within USATF. The previous CEO, Ollan Cassell, had usually participated in the work against doping, but his successor, Craig Masback, had a quite different approach. He defended one American athlete after another if they tested positive. Mary Decker-Slaney was the first.'

Inevitably, lawyers became involved. Proceedings commenced and would continue for years to come.

Masback, a lawyer by profession as well as a former international middle-distance runner, claimed that Slaney's drug test results were 'unclear', and that testosterone was difficult to detect in women.

'I've got no idea where he got that from. Testosterone is actually quite easy to test for in women. If there's any natural hormone that women have less of than men, then it is testosterone. Quite simply he didn't know what he was talking about.'

Annoyed that Slaney had been allowed to continue racing, even winning thousands of dollars in prize money at its own World Indoors in Paris, the IAAF decided soon afterwards to publicly suspend Slaney itself, thereby forcing USATF's hand.

The USATF reply was that Slaney was suffering from an endocrinological problem which explained why she had such high levels of testosterone.

'Naturally, we asked to see the evidence for this, but nothing ever turned up. Instead, USATF exonerated the athlete and lifted the suspension. The IAAF decided to send the case to the arbitration panel and a drawn-out process followed with incessant delays from the Americans. Finally the arbitration panel got tired of this and ruled in the absence of the Americans that Slaney was guilty of doping and it banned her for two years. Slaney continued to try to get her case tried in a civil court and the ruling overturned in the United States, but without success.'

There is a long list of other examples of how the USATF blocked the IAAF's ambitious anti-doping work around that period.

One example is the case of a world star who when he gave an adverse tests for elevated levels of testosterone, offered the explanation that he was HIV-positive and on the verge of developing Aids, and that was why his testosterone levels were so high.

It was a completely new medical phenomenon; of course, but the IAAF was forced to take the explanation seriously and examine the matter fully. 'I personally spoke on the telephone with his "doctor", who actually turned out not to be a doctor at all but a "trainer", or something along those lines. And they didn't want to send any proof that the athlete was HIV-positive. It was "personal".

'Back then the technology which can determine whether testosterone has been taken or is naturally elevated, didn't exist. Therefore, athletes with elevated testosterone levels were re-tested without warning. So we asked USATF to follow up the case. But nothing happened. In the end, they replied that the athlete had gone "underground": they couldn't find him. I then contacted IDTM, the agency we used to collect samples, who immediately sent out a doping control officer to the athlete's home address in America. When the doping control officer rang the door bell, the athlete opened the door.'

The athlete in question was banned for two years and disappeared from athletics.

Another example took place just when the conflict between the IAAF and USATF was about to reach its culmination, ahead of the 2000 Sydney Olympics. After the Decker-Slaney case, the IAAF took the view that USATF could not be trusted the next time an American tested positive. So before the Sydney Games, it was decided to ask for an overview of all positive results from every accredited doping lab.

The idea was to have everything cleared up before the Olympic Games. There were to be no cases that hadn't been resolved. That's why the IAAF even had its arbitration panel on hand in Sydney.

'Our inquiry to the laboratories was replied to very promptly with the exception of the lab in Indianapolis, which USATF used. We sent a reminder and received an answer saying that they had a shortage of staff because of economic difficulties. One day, IAAF doctor Gabriel Dolle rang me. We were both already in Sydney. He was upset. He had finally received the report from Indianapolis just before travelling to Sydney. It covered almost forty cases where athletes had tested positive but USATF had not reported to the IAAF as required by the rules, as the IAAF needs to be able to determine whether a case should be appealed or not.'

'This was dynamite so close to the Olympics and when the press found out, rumours began to spread. The big question, of course, was which American athletes who had failed drug tests were competing in Sydney.'

Arne understood that the newspapers, TV and radio wanted an immediate answer, but experience had taught him to keep the press at arm's length. 'I could barely leave my hotel room. There were journalists everywhere sensing catastrophe. I still didn't know any details myself, so I told them that the problem was the lack of information from the USTAF.'

At the same time, Gabriel Dolle met with Larry Bowers, the head of the Indianapolis laboratory. As it turned out, approximately half of the cases had either therapeutic exemptions for the substances involved, or there were other good reasons to set the case aside.

That left more than twenty athletes who had tested positive and had effectively been exonerated by their national governing body without the IAAF ever having been informed. 'I didn't know if any of them were in Sydney. That was the question the press wanted answered. I could only tell them to go and ask USATF and the US Olympic Committee. Of course, I put the same question to USATF myself, who denied that any of the athletes were in Sydney. That would turn out to be untrue.'

USATF was under a lot pressure. Lamine Diack, from Senegal, had only taken over as IAAF president in November 1999, following the death of Primo Nebiolo. In Sydney, with the Games opening ceremony just days away, Diack summoned Craig Masback to a meeting with Arne, Istvan Gyulai (the general secretary of the IAAF), and Bob Hersh (the US representative on the IAAF, and also a lawyer). And then it happened.

The American shot putter CJ Hunter suddenly called a press conference. Hunter, the world champion from 1999, had tested positive for the anabolic steroid Nandrolone earlier in the year after a competition in Oslo, Norway. The IAAF knew about the case, and was investigating it. USATF also knew about the positive test results, but they had still selected Hunter for the Sydney Olympics, apparently without informing the US Olympic Committee of the circumstances.

Hunter had his US team uniform and he had his Olympic accreditation and now suddenly he was giving a press conference, admitting through his tears that he had taken steroids over quite a period of time. Throughout the press conference, seated at his side, was Hunter's wife, Marion Jones.

Jones was probably the biggest world star in women's international athletics at the time. The 1997 and 1999 world champion at 100 metres, she was bidding in Sydney to win medals in five events – the 100 and 200 metres sprints, the long jump, and the 4x100 and 4x400 metres relays.

At the CJ Hunter press conference, she was tearful, too, but she managed to make a brief statement to the effect that she was entirely unaware that Hunter, the 330lb shot putter who was also her one-time strength and conditioning coach as well as her husband, had ever used banned drugs.

Soon after the press conference, Hunter was banned with immediate effect and he quit athletics. Eventually, Hunter and Jones were divorced.

Seven years later, Jones finally admitted that she, too, had doped.

'For us at the IAAF, it was a bit of a let-off that Hunter capitulated on his own accord. Plus that he did it just ahead of the Olympics.'

Yet still USATF dragged its feet. USATF maintained that American laws prohibited doping cases being made public before the case had been closed or dismissed, and that the same law prevented them from disclosing the identity of the athletes that they had exonerated.

'This was nonsense. They were just trying to sweep it all under the carpet and keep it all a secret. They lied to us straight in the face when they claimed it was against American law. To clear themselves they appointed their own commission to investigate the matter, led by Canadian professor of law Richard McLaren. His report was delivered in July 2001, and concluded that there was no American law prohibiting the reporting of doping cases to the IAAF, and that USATF's procedures were self-imposed restrictions that contravened the IAAF's rules and regulations.

'Furthermore, the McLaren Report revealed that one of the exonerated athletes had, indeed, competed in the Sydney Games. No name was given.

'Following the McLaren Report, we in the IAAF met with the USATF during the world championships in Edmonton in August 2001, in the hope that we could now move the matter forward. At the time, there must have been between thirteen and seventeen American doping cases that were unresolved and still of particular interest. But USATF told us that we would be allowed to review them only on an anonymous basis. We thought that such a review would be better than nothing. So we were very surprised and disappointed when they later told us that the US Olympic Committee would not allow that. Therefore, we met with the USOC president at the Salt Lake City Winter Olympics in February 2002. Contrary to what USATF had told us, the USOC had nothing against us reviewing the cases.

'By now, it was not only us at the IAAF who had had enough. Both the IOC and WADA presidents issued public statements in which the behaviour of the USATF was condemned.'

The driving force behind this campaign of secrecy was, as Arne understood it, Masback. Now, it seemed, with his position discovered, he switched tactics. 'In an interview in a journal, *The American Lawyer*, Masback claimed that

I was trying to push Lamine Diack to one side so I could take over the presidency of the IAAF. The claim lacked any credibility given that I was over seventy years old and wouldn't have had the energy to cope with that kind of responsibility.'

The only measure the IAAF could take against USATF was to expel them. That possibility was considered but in the end the IAAF turned to CAS. 'We asked two questions: A: did the IAAF have the right to get the information that was demanded?; and B: could USATF be forced to hand it over?

'If the answer was "yes" to the first question then logically it would also be for the second one. But that's not how it turned out.

'CAS answered "yes" to the first and "no" to the second question. By means of an explanation it was stated that the IAAF had not made it clear enough to the USATF which rules were being referred to in order to obtain the information. Furthermore, CAS stated that no athlete should be accused when he or she thinks that their case has been cleared up and resolved.'

The effect of the ruling was to place a time limit for the IAAF to investigate doping cases. USATF had been delaying and stalling on some of these cases since 1998.

'I can understand the second argument, but to set a period of limitation to just three years is far too little. The WADA Code now has an eight-year period of limitation.'

Arne believes in any case that CAS's argument was, in any case, wrong. On November 23, 1989, he had sent a letter to Ollan Cassell which contained an exact reference to the IAAF's regulations. Arne still has a copy of the letter, and he referred to it while questioned by CAS. The letter also formed part of the IAAF written submission to CAS.

'The letter is crystal clear proof that the IAAF acted correctly, and I was dismayed when CAS ignored its contents. It is not even mentioned in the judgement. The drawn-out conflict between the IAAF and USATF has been discussed in a book by WADA's first president, Dick Pound. He said that USATF "stonewalled the IAAF".'

THE CAS RULING did not mean an end to the affair, either. Indeed, it was quite the opposite.

USATF's persistent refusal to reveal which member of the American team at the Sydney Olympics had been identified by the McLaren Report as previously testing positive exasperated not just the IAAF and IOC but also many others, including American journalists. And it was one of these who eventually dug out the truth.

It was March 2002, and Arne held a press conference in New York after a scientific WADA symposium. 'A reporter from the *Los Angeles Times*, Alan Abrahamson, approached me.

'He had been looking into the American doping cases, and he had flown over to New York just to meet me. I can't reveal exactly what he told me. That's his affair. But the message was clear.

'He'd picked up on the scent and he wanted my reaction to what he had found out and hear my views before he went public.'

The story finally appeared in the pages of the *Los Angeles Times* on August 27, 2003. The athlete in question was 400-metre runner Jerome Young, who had run for the United States team in the heats of the 4x400 metres relay in Sydney, and had accordingly been presented with a gold medal when four of his team mates won the final.

Only after the intervention of the IOC, however, did the IAAF get hold of the necessary documents and so could examine the basis for USATF's earlier acquittal of Young.

Young had tested positive for the anabolic steroid Nandrolone in June 1999. Although the case was by now more than four years old, the IAAF ruled that Young's acquittal was without proper cause and appealed to CAS.

Another drawn-out legal case ensued, with written exchanges between CAS, the IAAF and USATF.

Eventually, CAS ruled in the IAAF's favour. 'Young was banned for two years, albeit retrospectively. We thought it would have some effect on the outcome of the relay race. The relay team was disqualified by the IAAF and just as the IOC was on the point of doing the same thing and taking back the gold medal for the Sydney Olympic Games from the Americans, USATF appealed to CAS.

'It seemed as if the case was going to go on forever. We thought that the disqualification was self-evident, but as it turned out CAS thought differently. It was claimed that IAAF's rules were unclear and the fact that Young did not participate in the final itself was sufficient reason not to disqualify the team in the final. This was in spite of them using a doped athlete to get to the final. But it was on this point that CAS thought that the IAAF's rules were insufficient.

'They turned a blind eye to any sporting sense of justice by ignoring the teams that did not field doped runners. So all the IAAF could do was go home and rewrite its rules.'

Yet even this wasn't the end of the case. In conjunction with a major investigation into doping in the United States, which would become known as the 'BALCO Scandal', a number of names were implicated as having doped, including participants in the team that competed in that 4x400 metres relay final in Sydney. One of them,

Antonio Pettigrew, admitted that he had been doping during the Sydney Olympic Games.

The WADA Code had extended the period of limitations on doping cases to eight years, and Pettigrew's admission occurred just before it expired for this case. On August 2, 2008, the IOC released a press statement which announced that Pettigrew was disqualified from his seventh place in the 400 metres final, and that the whole American relay team for the 4x400 metres at the Sydney Olympic Games was also disqualified and ordered to return their gold medals.

There was still more to come, though. In 2004, Young was handed a lifetime ban after he was caught doping for a second time, this time with EPO. And, at long last, Young admitted that he had been doping for most of his career, from 1991 to 2003. In February 2009, the IAAF announced that Young should be stripped of all the medals he had won at international competitions, including his individual 400 metres gold from the Paris world championships in 2003.

The Jerome Young case, which started with USATF trying to sweep everything under the carpet, had thus taken more than nine years to resolve. It had taken considerable effort and massive sums of money, and had even damaged CAS's reputation in the process.

Arne's dogged struggle against USATF's campaign of secrecy had long-term results. In 2000, Arne received a call from the White House. Support for his work had reached Presidential level.

Finally, America was to form an independent national anti-doping agency which was to take over anti-doping work from the US Olympic Committee. The so-called amateur sports in the United States, including USATF, lost all responsibility for handling doping matters. Instead it was handed over to a new, independent authority who received their budget direct from the US government.

Problems remained, however, within America's powerful, professional sports leagues, such as football and baseball. 'I had started my battle in the middle of the 1970s. Now, suddenly, it was part of major politics. Several years later, President George W Bush encouraged the heads of professional sport to take greater responsibility in the fight against doping. It was a crushing criticism of what hitherto looked like a systematic secrecy.'

America's new agency was named the United States Anti-Doping Agency, or USADA. It had actually been decided upon in 1999 and would soon be much talked about.

In 2003, with preparations for the 2004 Athens Olympics underway; the IAAF staged its world championships in Paris. 'The head of USADA, Terry Madden, called me and told me that the FBI had something massive going on involving the Justice Department. It was about some new kind of steroid that was being produced in huge quantities. It wasn't anything for which the world of sport had been testing.

'A coach had approached USADA with a syringe and told them that the substance it contained was being used by athletes. This is how the investigation had begun.

'Don Catlin, a member of the IOC's medical committee and head of the laboratory in Los Angeles, analysed the contents of the syringe. It was something called tetrahydrogestrinone, or THG for short, a "designer steroid" that had been created specifically to avoid detection in sports drug tests. It was untraceable with the current lab tests. What Madden told me was top secret. I couldn't even tell Diack.'

To ensure that nothing leaked until the FBI had sufficient material to make arrests, Arne and Terry Madden worked as 'secret agents'. The investigators supplied Arne with a list of those athletes who had been identified during the investigation. Arne then ordered doping tests through IDTM to be carried out on the non-American names on the list. USADA wanted to take care of the Americans. Only eight of the athletes on Arne's list were accessible.

Before the world championships started, Madden travelled to Paris and booked into a hotel a long way from the IAAF hotel or where the athletes were staying. He met Arne as well as the IAAF's lawyer, Huw Roberts. Larry Bowers, who had been head of the laboratory in Indianapolis and was now the scientific head of USADA, joined the meeting by telephone.

They had received information about BALCO – the Bay Area Laboratory Co-operative – an American company, based near San Francisco, which had produced supplements for athletes since 1988, but had long been suspected of supplying steroids to American bodybuilders and weightlifters. Now it was producing and supplying THG.

Not only had the drug been distributed to elite track athletes but also to sportsmen in the professional American sports leagues which, like bodybuilding, was not covered by any kind of anti-doping programme.

'There wasn't time or any possibility to go public with the information before the world championships, so I asked the head of the Paris lab to keep all the samples until further notice, including those that were negative. At the same time, I asked him not to ask me why. The intention, though, was to analyse them for the new steroid later on.'

It wasn't until the autumn of 2003 that the FBI was ready to move: an American company making 'undetectable' steroids for athletes. It was a massive scandal.

'But the results from the Paris world championships were scant. We only caught one athlete: Dwain Chambers, a British sprinter. He belonged to the small group that we had tested in the summer, just after we received the information about THG, and then again at the world championships. Both these tests were positive for THG. During the Athens Olympics the following year, we didn't find a single case of THG.'

Chambers made a comeback after having served his two-year disqualification, and in 2009 he published his memoirs in which he admits that he had been a customer of BALCO and used their products.

'The story of BALCO was a big thing in the media, but initially the identified athletes numbered just a few. It seemed for a while as if the whole thing had been blown out of proportion. But it was really because the wheels were turning slowly. Eventually, one big name after another became entangled in it: world record-holders like Tim Montgomery, and multiple medal-winners like Marion Jones. Proceedings are still going on and now include big names from Major League Baseball. It's awful to think that the athletes that took THG were actually like guinea pigs, testing it, perhaps even without understanding the dangers.

'THG had never gone through the stringent testing for effects and side-effects that a pharmaceutical drug must go through before it is put on the market. Here it was being given to elite sportsmen. It could have ended any way whatsoever. And we haven't seen the end of it yet.'

Chapter 13

More Lies, Cheating and Sabotage

ONE OF THE reasons for problems in handling matters involving the United States during the 1980s and 1990s was that the responsibility for anti-doping was divided between USA Track and Field and the United States Olympic Committee. When the IAAF complained that a doping case was handled incorrectly, or not handled at all, USATF and USOC usually blamed one another.

With the establishment of USADA, the situation improved considerably. Clearing up the BALCO scandal is just one example of how serious USADA is about its work. Arne was given specific details of the BALCO case in connection with the world championships in Paris in 2003.

And in Paris, another scandal took place which attracted much attention, and which ultimately would turn out to be linked to BALCO.

This case revolved around the winner of the women's sprint double, the American Kelli White. After one of her races she tested positive for Modafinil, a medication classified as a stimulant.

The world championships' sprint queen was doped – this was explosive stuff. 'Our problem was in classifying Modafinil. The substance wasn't on the list of banned substances but was a drug that gave you more energy and clearly came under the phrase "related substances" as part of the list of stimulants.

'The question was, however, if it should be regarded as a "strong" stimulant which would result in a two-year ban, or a "mild" stimulant that would only receive a warning. No matter what, she would be disqualified from the races and lose her gold medals. But I certainly needed to know ahead of the press conference that we were hastily forced to call: I knew it would be packed and there would be lots of questions.

'We consulted experts, who could not agree. Therefore we decided to treat Modafinil as a "mild" stimulant.'

In accordance with the usual protocols, White and her national association, USATF, were notified about the positive result and were asked to give an explanation. The answer was that White was suffering from narcolepsy – an unusual condition which means that you fall asleep without warning – and that she needed the stimulating medicine to keep her awake. A medical certificate was sent over and this made it apparent that it wasn't just White who suffered from it but that it was a hereditary illness within her family.

A Dr Goldman confirmed that he was treating Kelli and her family with Modafinil. A Therapeutic Use Exemption had not been requested as the substance was not on the list of banned substances. The doctor wrote to Arne arguing a case for why Modafinil should not be a banned substance. Clearly, the USATF campaign to clear White was underway.

But her appeal was rejected, Kelli White was disqualified and USATF was required to hand out a warning as the IAAF regulations stipulated.

Then something quite unexpected happened. While being questioned by the American authorities in conjunction with the BALCO case, Kelli White admitted that she had been one of BALCO's customers and had taken both Modafinil and other, even stronger doping substances.

'I had the occasion to meet her several years later, after I learned that Modafinil was part of BALCO's arsenal of doping drugs. I asked her how she and her family were doing with their narcolepsy.

'She smiled and said that she had never suffered from it and neither had her family. Nor had she ever met Dr Goldman who wrote her the falsified medical certificate. I've been assured that he was struck off for a period of time, but I don't know how long. Kelli White was banned for two years and has not returned to competitive athletics since.'

THE WHOLE BALCO story broke just ahead of the Athens Olympics, but the 2004 Games already had a doping scandal hanging around its neck. This involved two of the host nation's best hopes of medals in track and field – the sprinters Kostas Kenteris and Ekaterina Thanou.

'We really sharpened up in Athens. It was the Olympics that we covered the best until then. We had introduced something called "the Olympic period", which ran from when the Olympic Village opened to the close of the Games. During this time, all the participants were required to be available for testing under the Olympic rules.'

In the week before the Games began, Kenteris, the reigning Olympic 200 metres champion, was widely expected to be involved in lighting the Olympic flame at the Opening Ceremony, which as usual would be staged nearly a week before the first athletics events would get underway. Both Kenteris and Thanou had given their whereabouts as Chicago, so WADA sent doping control officers there.

When the testers got there, it turned out that the sprinters had in fact gone to Germany. The staff from WADA tried to track them down, but they soon found that they weren't in Germany, either.

'I was kept informed about the attempts to find the two athletes. I feared that this could become an enormously embarrassing story, particularly for our Greek hosts. Then one day I got a phone call.

'The two of them had apparently turned up at the Olympic Village. We could test them there. In the evening, the phone rang again. Kenteris and Thanou had been in the Village but had now moved on again. No one knew where they were. There hadn't been enough time to test them.

'Clearly, they had been tipped off or knew that doping control officers were looking for them. We reported the matter to the IOC's head of disciplinary matters, as it really looked like they were avoiding being tested, which is itself an offence.

'A new report then turned up from the Greeks. Kenteris and Thanou had been involved in a motorcycle accident and now were in hospital. They were hurt but only suffering minor injuries. The report stated that they would soon be able to leave the hospital and the IOC called them in for questioning the next day.

'A letter then came from their doctors, saying that they could not be released yet. They required two more days in hospital. The IOC postponed the hearing by seventy-two hours to give them a bit of leeway. And that's how it carried on. We held off and the doctors delayed things.

'Eventually, a week had passed and we declared that this was enough so then they turned up. Without comment, they just handed in their Olympic accreditation. In doing so, they were no longer under the jurisdiction of the IOC and could not participate in the Olympics.

'The matter was then passed to the IAAF to be dealt with after the Games. After more lengthy procedures, they were banned for two years. In January 2011 it was reported that the prosecution would start on the basis of the athletes having faked the motorcycle accident.'

Thanks to the intensive drug testing at the Games, the doping findings for Athens were considerably higher than for Sydney four years earlier. Ten cases of doping were caught in Sydney, compared to sixteen in Athens.

At the same time as reliable methods of analysis were being developed, the legal framework developed. The WADA Code from 2004 and the UNESCO convention from 2007 were decisive milestones. But they didn't prevent sportsmen and women from initiating expensive legal proceedings at CAS.

One case in point is Floyd Landis, the American cyclist and Tour de France winner who, in 2008, appealed to CAS against being disqualified for testosterone doping. The international cycling federation could not afford to defend the charge, so WADA stepped in to their place. The disqualification was upheld, but the case cost WADA between US$1.5 and $2 million, almost thirty per cent of WADA's annual research budget. And in May 2010 Landis admitted having doped.

But there are examples of how even greater sums have been involved. 'The case of Harry "Butch" Reynolds is a clear example of this and one of the most spectacular sporting trials in our history.

'Reynolds was superb at the 400 metres, held the world record and was ranked world No. 1 when he was found to have Nandrolone in his body in 1990. Initially everything went as it should, and the American federation banned him. Then it started. Reynolds found a legal loophole and had the ban overturned by the appeals board of the American association. Certain procedural mistakes were alleged.

'The IAAF took the matter to the arbitration panel, who concurred with Reynolds that the rules had not been followed to the letter, but at the same time maintained that this had not affected his urine sample. Reynolds was still guilty of doping.

'This was an important precedent. It's not enough to show that there are weaknesses in the procedure; you have to be able to prove that it influenced the result of the drug test.'

Reynolds' lawyer wouldn't give up. They took the matter to the American courts. At home in Akron, Ohio, they put the case before an eighty-seven-year-old judge who cleared Reynolds and ordered the IAAF to pay the ludicrous amount of US$27.4 million in compensation. To secure the fine, the judge ordered that the IAAF's assets in the United States should be frozen.

The ruling was overturned by a court at the next level, a circular court, which ruled that the civil legal system had no jurisdiction in the case. And when Reynolds' lawyer took the case further, to the US Supreme Court, they refused to try the case.

It was apparent that the American legal system respected that sport should be allowed to govern itself and rule on matters such as this.

Trials like the one with Reynolds are not just drawn-out, they are also expensive, even if they don't result in the IAAF having to pay damages. Each case that goes to the arbitration panel costs the IAAF between US$100,000 and US$150,000, whatever the outcome. The only people guaranteed a profit from the trials are the lawyers who scrutinise the rules, hunting for loopholes so they can claim damages for their clients.

'One example of how an apparently simple matter can unexpectedly become complicated with dramatic consequences, and a potential matter for the arbitration panel, is the case of Diane Modahl, the British middle-distance runner who won gold at the Commonwealth Games in Auckland, New Zealand in 1990, but had an adverse test for testosterone in a drug test conducted after she had raced in Portugal early in the 1994 season.

'Her national governing body, then called the British Athletics Federation, convicted her of doping, but Modahl got in touch with someone called Simon Gaskell, who was meant to be some kind of expert. Gaskell argued that there could have been a degradation of the urine sample if it had been contaminated by bacteria. He claimed that this was what had happened since the sample had been left in room temperature for some time.

'It was not possible to prove or disprove this. There are methods to see if testosterone developed in the sample after it had been taken, but no such analysis had been done; so when we came to decide whether the matter should be passed to the arbitration panel following her successful appeal in Britain, it turned out that we lacked sufficient grounds. We had no other choice than to let the case rest, which resulted in the British federation being sued by Modahl for having convicted her in the first instance. They were hit with such massive damages that the federation went bust.'

More Lies, Cheating and Sabotage

THERE ARE ALSO examples of casuistry which are not just drawn-out and expensive, but totally extraordinary, even sensational, even if they never reach the back pages of the world's newspapers or the television bulletins. Arne has kept notes about one especially unusual, cynical and bizarre case.

A Russian participant at the 1999 world championships in Seville tested positive for hCG – Human chorionic gonadotropin. HCG can have a doping effect by stimulating the body's own production of testosterone. It is also used by those who are doping with testosterone: long-term misuse of testosterone can suppress the body's own production of the hormone and in worst cases make the doper's testosterone levels so low that the body even ceases to produce any. When this happens, hCG is therefore taken at intervals to stimulate the body's own production of testosterone.

From a sporting perspective, using hCG is regarded equally to using anabolic steroids, and its use incurs a two-year ban.

'When we caught him with this substance in his body we contacted his national athletics federation and asked for an explanation. They replied that the athlete was suffering from a problem with his prostate.'

There were two things that were odd about this explanation. First, the athlete was too young to have prostate problems, with the possible exception of prostatitis. 'Perhaps most importantly though, hCG has nothing to do with the prostate.

'So we informed the Russian federation that we considered it a case of doping until further notice. We then received a new message: now he had a kidney problem. Perhaps that was the cause of his increased level of hCG? When we didn't accept that explanation either, as it didn't hold scientifically, we received a third letter claiming it was now a problem to do with his testicles. It didn't go into details, but I knew there is an exceedingly malignant and unusual testicular cancer that really can cause the body to produce hCG. It is ordinarily produced by pregnant women in the placenta, but testicular germ cells may develop a rare form of cancer which exhibit signs of being placenta-like in character. But the third letter didn't mention cancer, just testis inflammation.'

The matter remained a case of doping as far as the IAAF was concerned. Then a fourth letter arrived from the Russians confirming he was suffering from testicular cancer and that he was terminally ill. The IAAF, they said, ought to leave him in peace.

The athlete had had a testicle surgically removed and he was undergoing chemotherapy.

'I was suspicious and I asked to examine a sample from the removed testicle under microscope. I have analysed and diagnosed cancer for forty years, so this is something I know. I received microscopic slides and a signed statement which described the nature of the tumour. The only problem was that the stated diagnosis of a Leydig cell tumour, which was correct in accordance with the microscopic slides, had nothing to do with the production of hCG.

'The case was now into its second year. However, the athlete's national federation wouldn't give up. They stated that he had a different type of cancer. Apparently, the samples had been mixed up at the hospital where he had undergone surgery.'

Arne now received what was said to be the correct slides with the newly signed doctor's certificate. Now it really was a case of choriocarcinoma. 'I'd had enough and contacted the president of the IAAF, Lamine Diack. We suggested an independent examination of the athlete in Sweden. Until this point, we had only received a stream of weird diagnoses and woolly explanations.'

The Russians rejected the notion of an independent examination, again on the basis that the athlete was too ill to be moved. Diack then gave them an ultimatum: they had to accept the examination or the case would be turned over to CAS, the Court for Arbitration in Sport.

It was then that the Russians gave up. A message arrived which said that the athlete had been banned for two years. 'But how can you ban someone so sick and suffering from cancer at the same time as claiming that the test results were a result of the illness?' I asked the president of the Russian federation the next occasion that I met him. I was given a wry smile as an answer.'

When his two-year ban was completed, the athlete who had been said to be so sick with cancer turned up and started competing again with some success, including at the 2003 world championships in Paris. 'Then we got hold of him and could finally examine how he, who so recently had been terminally ill with cancer, could compete at an elite level. He willingly let himself be examined. We couldn't find any trace of an operation. He had two completely normal testes.

'I realised he had probably been completely in the dark about the game that had gone on.'

THE RUSSIANS DISTINGUISHED themselves again at the Beijing Olympic Games in 2008.

In the months leading up to the Olympics, the IAAF had noticed that it was very easy to get out-of-competition tests carried out on elite Russian athletes and that there was almost never a problem with their whereabouts reports. It all looked too good to be true.

So an investigation was ordered. For more than a year before Beijing, urine samples taken from some elite athletes in out-of-competition tests were compared with those taken at different competitions. DNA analysis was used, revealing that the urine provided by the athletes at their out-of-competition tests did not match the DNA in the urine samples from the same athletes taken at the competitions. They were using someone else's urine.

This dramatic development, the result of sixteen months of painstakingly careful work by the IAAF, was announced just before the Olympic Games in Beijing and seven Russian women, five of them in the Olympic team – including Yelena Soboleva, then the world indoor champion at 1,500 metres, and Tatyana Tomashova, the 2004 Olympic silver medal-winner at 1,500 metres – were immediately suspended for having manipulated their tests. They never went to Beijing.

AT A PRESS conference in Beijing, Arne described what had happened as 'organised and systematic doping ... taking place within Russian sport'. The remark was not popular in Russia.

But Arne soon received support for his statement. Before the biathlon world championships had begun in PyeongChang in South Korea in February 2009, three more Russian stars were sent home having tested positive earlier in the season for a variant of EPO, the hormone which stimulates the production of red blood cells, thus increasing stamina.

Anders Besseberg, the international biathlon federation's chairman, who is also on the board of WADA, now came forward to make a public statement condemning the systematic doping being carried out by Russian biathletes.

It is not just in the United States and Russia that a culture of doping thrives in sport. The entire former Eastern bloc has continued to be a problem since the downfall of the Soviet Union. Among the seven athletes who tested positive during the Beijing Olympics were two Belorussian hammer throwers (later exonerated by CAS for technical reasons), a Ukrainian heptathlete and a Polish canoeist. Every case involved steroids. For the Ukrainian woman, it was the second time in her career which meant a lifetime ban.

But even in other parts of the world there is a problem. One notable case was revealed at the Winter Olympics in Turin in 2006. Here, Arne found himself in the role of the chief detective in a crime story rather than a doctor at a sporting event.

'It was a couple of days after I arrived in Turin that I learned that WADA had attempted to carry out an out-of-competition drugs test on the Austrian cross-country skiing and biathlon teams before they set off for Turin. According to the official whereabouts report that WADA had received, the skiers should have been stationed at a training camp in Austria. But when the doping control officers arrived at the given address, a guest house, no skiers were there.

'However, in the guest house's cellar they found what looked like a haematological laboratory. It really *felt* of blood doping. The doping control officers were quickly ushered away by the owner of the guest house, who turned out to be the wife of the Austrian ski trainer Walther Maier – the same Walter Maier who had received an unprecedented ten-year ban from the IOC at Salt Lake City four years earlier, when he had been found with an array of transfusion equipment which suggested that he was tampering with the blood of the Austrian ski team.

'On that occasion, no active skier had been caught testing positive.

'But this time, news came through that Walther Maier had been spotted in the Turin area, in the vicinity of the Austrian camp, even though he was not accredited by the Olympics. As Italy has a very strict doping law, and doping offences can be treated as criminal offences, we felt obliged to inform our Italian hosts.'

On the morning of Thursday February 16, a meeting was held in the hotel suite of IOC President Jacques Rogge. Present was Rogge, Arne and two other representatives from the IOC, together with the Italian sports minister and the chief of the Italian anti-doping organisation. The IOC-delegation handed over to the Italians the information that they had got from WADA, then outlined their own observations about Maier's presence and revealed that they intended to carry out a surprise test of the Austrian cross-country skiers and biathletes on Saturday evening.

'We were forced to give the Italians some time to consider the information. At the same time, I was scared that something would be leaked giving the Austrians time to prepare before Saturday evening. Perhaps they would make themselves unavailable.

'But the Italians kept quiet. They got back to us on Saturday morning and informed us that they regarded the case as so serious that they were thinking about raiding the Austrian camp. They suggested that we should co-ordinate a raid that evening.'

Arne found himself heading the investigation with a group of 'troops'. The IOC's doping control officers and the *carabinieri*, set off at the same time for the Austrian camps in Sestriere and Pragelato. Apart from a few red traffic lights that slowed them down, it went like clockwork, with both raids happening simultaneously.

There was panic in the Austrian camp. Medical instruments and other material were thrown out the window and the Austrians tried to get away. Walter Maier disappeared in his car towards the Austrian border, but was stopped at a police roadblock. He ended up in hospital, apparently with excessive alcohol in his blood.

Two biathletes returned home to Austria, from where they announced their immediate retirement. Several other Austrian skiers and biathletes were tested.

The events made big news. Arne was forced to hold a press conference and explain what had happened. He was fiercely questioned, especially by the Austrian media. More press conferences took place. The Italians didn't say much about what had happened, but Arne was forced to admit at a press conference that all the drug tests had proved negative.

'It wasn't that surprising. They had, of course, planned the tampering with their blood so it would test negative at the upcoming events. But we were forced to act as we did. At the press conference, I was sarcastically asked by Austrian journalists why I had made such a fuss: everyone was negative, so it wasn't doping, they said.

'I replied that doping is not just about testing positive. For example, there's possessing doping medication and doping equipment.'

There was a long wait for the report from the Italians. The matter had ended up on the desk of Turin's notoriously aggressive public prosecutor, Raffaele Guarinielli. 'I visited Guarinielli in Turin. He was a friendly but very determined gentleman. We were in contact for a long time!'

As late as October 2008, Guarinielli gave notice that he intended to charge a long list of Austrian officials and athletes for breaking Italy's doping laws. But before this, the IOC received enough information from Guarinielli confirming that blood doping equipment had been found, as well as banned doping substances in the Austrian camp. It was sufficient for the IOC to act.

Several cross-country skiers as well as team managers were banned from competing in future Olympics. The Austrian Olympic Committee was fined a US$1 million by the IOC for failing to monitor its team sufficiently. The international ski federation banned the athletes in question and the team leaders for two years. Some of the athletes appealed to CAS against their conviction, without success. In June 2009, the Italian prosecutors indicted ten Austrian officials and skiers for having violated the Italian doping law.

'Sure, it was a successful case. Internally, we referred to it with a touch of gallows humour as "Operation Sachertarte"*, but the Austrians probably don't like that.

'It's really tragic for sport that something like this needs to happen. At the same time the events are a good example of having an effective law in place in the country that is arranging a major international event. It was because they had the law on their side that the Italians could carry out such a raid and find what they did. If the Italian anti-doping law hadn't existed, the cheating being done by the Austrians would never have been discovered. All the tests were negative, after all.

'At the IOC session in Guatemala in June 2007, I met the Austrian premier, Alfred Gusenbauer. He was there because Salzburg was a candidate to host the 2014 Winter Olympics, but he wanted to meet me. I felt a little embarrassed and apologised a bit for what we had done in Turin.

'But he wanted to thank me for the effective action we had taken which had revealed the unacceptable cheating. It had made it possible for the Austrian parliament to pass a law in record time with strong anti-doping rules.'

* Sachertarte is a Viennese cake.

Chapter 13

Women, Gender Testing and the Dangers of Elite Sport

SPORT IS PART of society. It reflects the society it takes place in, and is characterised by its values – whether good or ill. Doping in sport is an example of this, both the work against drug-use as well as the propagation of doping itself. Sex-discrimination and bullying are also part of society, and therefore of sport. Both still occur, even though they are banned by law.

Sport in Sweden tries to combat any form of unfair treatment. Work is still going on to formulate a policy, developing action plans and trying to change attitudes. The Swedish Sports Confederation's plan of action against sexual harassment defines the phenomenon as follows:

An unwelcome approach of a sexual nature which infringes upon girls and boys, women and men, who actively compete, volunteer or are employed within sport.

The most important characteristic of harassment is that it is unwanted by the person subject to it. The decisive factor is how the individual subjected to harassment experiences it, and not the motives of the person harassing them.

Arne sees the position thus: 'So the Swedish Sports Confederation has declared its standpoint and developed a plan of action. This can serve as a basis for other countries. The IOC recently presented a similar plan. These are questions we simply cannot close our eyes to, and within the IOC medical committee's working group, we are constantly striving to combat sexual harassment in sport.

'The working group is made up of experts from the whole world: doctors, psychologists, counsellors and psychiatrists working to prevent problems. We're between fifteen and twenty people in total collaborating on the plan of action, documenting these kinds of questions and producing educational material.'

But such issues are not going to be solved by policy documents or legal legislation. This is a problem that occurs between people in sport. It's often about coaches and trainers who often have a grip on their young protégés. It's about male coaches and trainers, and girls and women. Between the young and old. Young boys are also vulnerable, as well-known cases in a range of sports have illustrated.

It's the coaches and trainers themselves who are finally answerable for their actions. 'It is the responsibility of each and every one of them to ensure that no one is subject to harassment.'

THERE WAS A systematic violation, for which the world of sport must take responsibility, that took place over the course of many years under the name of 'gender testing'. A gender certificate issued by sports authorities was required in order to compete in women's events.

'There's not many who know about this humiliating chapter of the history of sport, other than those who were affected by it. It seems that the media never realised the extent to which gender testing took place, or perhaps didn't care about it.

'It took a long battle to put an end to gender testing. This was a decades-long example of sexual harassment within sport. Gender testing was a flagrant abuse, nothing else.'

The history of gender testing goes back to the 1960s. There had been rumours for years that there were athletes competing in the women's events who were more male than female, making it an unfair competition for 'real' women.

To thwart the rumours, the IOC decided to introduce some kind of control. 'Sport had no other means of asserting the gender of participants other than having them parade naked in front of a panel of doctors. After this "examination", the panel decided whether the case presented to them was a woman or a man.'

Gender testing of this type was introduced for the first time at athletics' European Championships in Budapest in 1966.

This kind of examination was replaced with a laboratory method of testing gender, the 'buccal smear test'. Cells were scraped from inside the competitor's mouth and analysed to establish if their chromosomes were male or female. This method of testing was introduced at the Olympics in 1968. The programme was led by a male Mexican gynaecologist and was allowed to continue long into the 1980s without any change or questioning about its ethics or efficacy. The media remained quiet about this, along with the competitors and public.

Despite the gender tests, the malicious rumours about some masculine-looking sportswomen, which the tests were introduced to end, continued. But sports officials seemed satisfied that the tests guaranteed that only women competed in women's events. At least, they did until the 1985 Universiade – World University Games – in Kobe, Japan.

Every athlete who successfully passed the gender test received a certificate stating her gender, and did not need to go through the test again when competing in the future

One of the competitors in Kobe was Maria Patino, Spain's leading sprint hurdler. In 1983, she had gone through gender testing at the world championships in Helsinki and got her certificate to 'prove' she was a woman.

But when she arrived in Kobe, Patino realised that she had left her certificate at home in Spain, so she had to take another gender test. When the results came through, it showed that she had male chromosomes. The laboratory result completely contradicted the results of her first gender test.

Patino was not allowed to compete in Japan, and her national federation tried to persuade her not to race again. However, the result of her gender test was leaked to the Spanish press. There was uproar. Patino had to face the full glare of the media, she was dropped by the Spanish athletics federation, she lost her university scholarship, and even her boyfriend left her. At twenty-four, her life was in tatters.

Yet against all odds, Patino managed to pick herself up to question what had happened to her. She contacted a professor in clinical genetics in Helsinki, Albert de la Chapelle, who she knew was opposed to gender testing.

'Albert and I knew each other from evaluating applications at the Karolinska Institutet. We got on well, sharing each other's point of view, even if others didn't. We were kindred spirits.

'So Albert rang me as he knew I was involved in the running of international athletics. He explained what the problem was, and I understood the dilemma. I asked myself what on earth the world of sport was doing? We were both in agreement that gender tests were completely unscientific. That was true in 1968 and damn well wasn't it 1985!'

The previous two decades had seen techniques developed and a greater understanding about sex chromosomes and how they affect a person's gender. By 1985, science knew that it wasn't simply the sex chromosomes that determined if you were a man or a woman. 'There are women with a male set of chromosomes and vice versa, as well as a whole host of variations in between. The thinking upon which the gender tests were based when they were introduced in the 1960s was antiquated by 1985. Besides, as the case of the Spanish hurdler demonstrated, the actual method of analysis was unreliable.

'I took up the case and again there was a massive uproar. After nearly three years, Patino was reinstated. She became my eternal supporter. She is now a respected university lecturer in sports education at Galicia in Spain and she still keeps in touch by letter, email or phone. We have even written a scientific article regarding gender testing together.'

For Arne, the Patino case was just the start of yet another battle. 'I wanted to persuade the IAAF and IOC to stop this idiocy.'

The first thing Arne did was to invite Albert de la Chapelle to the scientific symposium that the IAAF held in Canberra, Australia, in conjunction with the World Cup in 1985. He let Chapelle explain the genetic situation for the gathered leaders of sport and sports medicine experts. The IAAF was positive about making changes, but gender testing did not cease in athletics until the beginning of the 1990s. 'It just shows how long it can take to change something. You have to create a flow of information and generate opinion. After that, it's only the federation's congress that can change the sport's rules, and the IAAF only holds a congress every other year.'

Within the IOC the situation was completely different. 'Prince Alexandre de Mérode was the chairman of the IOC's medical committee.

During the mid-1960s, as a relatively new member of the IOC, he was handed the task of developing the medical committee after Knud Jensen's death at the 1960 Rome Games. The committee's main duty was to stem drug abuse, but in 1968 it had got wind of this method of guaranteeing that girls were indeed girls. Prince de Mérode thought it was a splendid idea and he supported it.

'In most ways, we got on very well, he and I, and he was clever in many ways, but we clashed over this. The prince certainly wasn't a doctor, he had no scientific training, and it proved impossible to get him to understand that gender testing was ridiculous. I tried in every way possible to convince him, but it was completely impossible. We didn't stand a chance of changing things while de Mérode remained in office.'

Arne didn't give up. With the help of other opponents to gender testing within the IOC, and using public opinion, he built up a campaign against the tests. When it was strong enough, it would at least be embarrassing for de Mérode.

Meanwhile, scientific knowledge was increasing. An improved method of analysing sex chromosomes was launched for the 1992 Winter Olympics in Albertville. 'Prince de Mérode still didn't want to understand that it wasn't the method of analysis that was the problem. It is much more complicated than that. It is the very ideology behind the tests.

'It was very clear now, however, that this was a matter of prestige for him. In Nagano in 1998, an American journalist picked up on the issue. She was interested in what was going to happen ahead of the Salt Lake City Winter Games in 2002. It was only then that it started to get picked up by the international press. She called my work "a one man crusade", and in her opinion I was doomed to failure because the chairman of the IOC's medical committee was against me, as was the only woman on the board of the IOC, the vice-president, Anita de Frantz, from the United States.'

Eventually, even de Mérode began to get uneasy about the whole thing. He arranged for a conference on the subject, with the objective of picking holes in Arne's argument. He invited all kinds of scientists who had been involved in developing the refined chromosome-defining method and had worked with the programme after Albertville. 'They missed the point that it wasn't about it being the wrong kind of technique, but that gender cannot be determined purely by laboratory analysis. Again it resulted in nothing.'

Arne then managed to persuade the IOC's athletes' commission to act. Arne and the commission's chairman, Peter Tallberg, from Finland, agreed that the commission should highlight the issue and give the IOC board a recommendation. On the commission was Johan Olav Koss. Many people remember him as an outstanding speed skater from the 1994 Olympics in Lillehammer, but he had also studied medicine even though he wasn't yet a fully qualified doctor.

'Koss was a good friend of mine and he was asked to be responsible for investigating the question of gender testing on behalf of the commission. Peter Tallberg and I reckoned that if the athletes' commission arrived at the decision that gender testing should be stopped, the IOC's board would hardly be able to object. I supplied Koss with all the arguments against the gender-testing programme, together with the documentation, articles and scientific background. I also consulted with Albert de la Chapelle and several other leading international scientists within the field.

'Johan incorporated all my arguments and my material into the commission's work, made an independent analysis of them and had them evaluated by even more experts. Finally, at the end of 1998, the commission put forward its recommendations to the IOC.

'The commission called upon the IOC to stop the degrading gender tests.'

Finally the IOC capitulated under the pressure, just as Arne and his working group had hoped when they had first set out their strategy. But de Mérode remained chairman of the IOC's medical committee and retained his position of power within the IOC. Accordingly, as a gesture, they announced that the gender tests would cease on a trial basis at the 2000 Sydney Olympic Games.

Behind the scenes, another game was also going on. Jacques Rogge would soon be standing for the position of IOC President. Rogge was a doctor and well understood Arne's position. But like de Mérode, he was also a Belgian.

'It was crystal clear that there was rivalry between them. But I knew that Rogge supported me, and that was enough. This was still under Samaranch's presidency and I had certainly indoctrinated him to understand the matter, but he found it hard to take up the battle. Juan Antonio Samaranch was afraid of conflict. Of course, this didn't stop me from raising the matter, and after fifteen years I got what I wanted. The IOC did away with the compulsory gender testing of all female Olympians, and in the early 2000s the international federations followed suit. Today, investigation of an athletes' gender occurs rarely, and only if there is a reason for it'

IT IS EASY when discussing sport and doping to get the impression that the latter is the only threat against the athlete's health. Or the idea that all sport, if you just keep away from drugs and banned substances, is good for your health. But that's not the entire story.

Many children are attracted to sport. It is similar to playing games. In the past there was even a subject at school in Sweden called 'Games and Sport'. As they get older, some children drift away from games at school. Some are better than others at sport, depending on a whole range of influences, such as genetic factors, environment and diet. A few are so good at their chosen sport that they are recruited by clubs who invest in them by providing trainers and coaches. But eventually, only a very few go on and decide to aim for a career in elite sport.

'In connection with this I think it is appropriate and about time to demand that the world of sport takes more responsibility for the young people it recruits. This is because the world of sport has both a moral and medical responsibility.

'We have not been good enough at telling those who want to aim for a career in elite sports what it actually entails. Elite sports entail massive effort and risks. Yes, very real medical risks that in the worst of cases can lead to life-long health problems.

'We need to impress upon them even more clearly that an elite athlete certainly strengthens his or her body; nonetheless, he or she also puts it under an enormous strain.

'The health benefits of being an elite athlete can never be used to entice young people or persuade them to embark on an elite career. You have to understand that you are putting yourself at risk by playing sport at an elite level, although it does have other great benefits.

'On the IOC's medical committee we have, under my stewardship, raised these questions for discussion. We're working quite differently since the anti-doping issues were handed over to WADA. Now the committee has time to work with other issues: this is one of the things we're engaged in. It's our responsibility to reduce injuries and illness within elite sport, I think, and now we have produced information material, recommendations and policy documents. Our overriding motto is: "The protection of the health of the athlete".'

A while ago the committee outlined its general position and programme to combat anorexia within sport. This move echoes the response of shocked audiences who've seen so many emaciated athletes at sports stadiums But it takes time to change big issues. 'To get some kind of result, statement and programme, we sought the help of some of the world's leading experts as we realised that there was an over-representation of the illness amongst elite athletes.

'We have also developed a programme against what we call "sudden death in sport" – when young athletes, at the peak of their fitness, drop down dead while participating in sporting events. We have also looked at different kinds of injuries that occur in conjunction with sport such as concussion or accidents in skiing and football, and we have also looked at how elite sport affects children and young people.

'I believe that moderate exercise and sport is good for your health, but the health benefits of sport cannot be used as a motivation for doing it at an elite level. There are other benefits at that level.'

Chapter 14

Clubs and Societies

MEMBERS OF THE council of the IAAF serve for four years at a time. In 2007, Arne's eighth mandate period expired. He had to decide between stepping down or taking on a ninth term on the council. If he accepted, he would reach eighty years of age before he could step down, and he had already served on the board for more than thirty years. Arne decided to step down. 'I felt like I had done my bit after so many years. More than most at the top of international sport.

'The first person who got to know how I was thinking was the IAAF president, Lamine Diack. He didn't try and convince me otherwise, but simply said: "We have to talk." So he got on a plane to Stockholm. I picked him up and drove him home to Enebyberg, and there we sat and talked for many hours. We talked about what had happened, and what was going to happen in the future. He asked me if he could use me as a sounding board, and of course I agreed. We both joined the IAAF at the same time and have known each other over all these years. Lamine was there and thanked me for my services when my resignation was made public in July 2007 at the IOC session in Guatemala. I was then acclaimed and thanked for my services once again during the world championships in Osaka later in the year when I also received the IAAF's Golden Order of Honour.

'Obviously, when you leave a post such as this you really miss it. But it was nice to know that I had so much support, and most of all those people felt that I still had much to give when I stepped down. I was very relieved when I made my decision. It was agony deciding, even though I made the right decision.'

FOR DECADES, ARNE has been one of the outstanding officials in the world of sport. Throughout his career as a doctor, professor, researcher and opinion-maker he has taken on doping. At the same time, he had been Sweden's face in the world of international athletics. There is no one who has taken on that role after him.

It was in Stockholm in 1912 that the IAAF was founded. The first president was a Swede, and so was the secretary, treasurer and several other members. Except for a ten-year period straight after the Second World War, there has always been a Swede on the Council of the IAAF. Until now, that is.

Today the federation has more than two hundred member countries. The council has just twenty-six members. That Sweden should have a guaranteed post on the council is by no means self-evident. Not to anyone around the world or even in Sweden. The lack of understanding in Sweden that the country needs to take care of its position internationally is astonishing to Arne. 'There is no Swede left today on the council of a federation founded in Sweden. It's not just unfortunate, it's bad management on our part.

'The reason isn't that I've sat there blocking others from coming forward. It's been exactly the opposite. I have continually tried to persuade the head of the Swedish federation to recruit someone who could take over after me, but I haven't got any response. They've been completely uninterested over the years; I would say they haven't even cared.

'This is probably because there is a lack of understanding for how important it is for Sweden to be a part of the decision-making bodies that govern international sport. I've tried to work on my successors as federation president, but no one has listened or realised the significance of the issue.'

Arne did his best to try to recruit a successor. He asked Yngve Andersson, who has recently stepped down as federation president, but he wasn't interested in an international career. One possible candidate was the secretary general for the 2006 European Championships staged in Gothenburg, Toralf Nilsson, but around the same time he was elected to the board of the European Athletic Association, which in itself was good.

Another suitable candidate, Arne felt, was Rajne Söderberg, head of the annual DN-Gala grand prix event staged in Stockholm and, like Arne, also a doctor.

Rajne works within the world of sport and has a network of contacts like very few others. There was only one thing in his way. The IAAF stipulates that candidates have to be proposed by their national athletics association. Rajne Söderberg wasn't a member. 'So I suggested to Yngve Andersson that Rajne ought to stand for election to the board of the Swedish federation in 2004, so he could go on to become Sweden's international representative. But the election committee opposed this and selected another candidate.

'You have to wonder what were they thinking? Are we just meant to sit and play in our own sandpit? Don't those who govern Swedish athletics realise that sport is being internationalised? Given that our athletes were so successful, shouldn't we also be part of the international organisation that governs sport?

'I had to postpone promoting Rajne until 2006. I pushed more this time and finally the election committee grasped how important this was and proposed him. When he still wasn't elected by the general assembly, I gave up.'

TO KEEP BEING involved in a mission can easily become something of an end in itself if you stay involved for too long. To that end, Arne has on principal always declared how long he intended to remain in a post before he took one up. His post at the IAAF is the biggest exception to the rule. Still, it was natural that he eventually stepped aside. Even so, he knew that he wanted to concentrate on tackling the issues he believed were most urgent, and the major factor that persauded him to leave the IAAF was that he was nominated for the post of vice-president of WADA.

The running and financing of WADA is divided equally between the governments around the world and the Olympic movement. The presidency of WADA is given to a government representative for one mandate period and is then followed by a sporting representative. And when the governments have the presidency, the vice-president is an Olympic movement representative, and vice versa. The election of Arne as vice-president in 2007 made him world sport's highest representative within the fight against doping.

'When I heard that I had been nominated I talked to Jacque Rogge, president of the IOC. "My dear," I said, "at my age!" Rogge said that I ought best to accept the post. The entire world of sport supported me. There weren't any alternative candidates.' Arne took the decision to leave the IAAF before the WADA nomination was made public. The reason wasn't just personal and it wasn't just about the years and years that he had served the IAAF.

'It is also because WADA has a supervisory responsibility over the international federations. There would be a risk that there would be a conflict of interests if I was on the board of one federation and WADA's simultaneously. I didn't want that.'

How is it that Arne Ljungqvist gets one job after another, goes from one board to another? Is it luck? Or skill? Or a matter of circumstance?

Perhaps it is a bit of all at once. But Sweden is also a country where there are lots of clubs and societies. Within every part of public life clubs and societies thrive. And Arne is a child of his nation. There is a particular word for it in Swedish: *föreningsmänniskor.* Someone who likes belonging to clubs and societies.

Arne is one such person. And perhaps he is one of those who has gone the furthest in his engagement in clubs and societies. It feels like he loves to lead a meeting or take charge of things for the board. He is incredibly good at it too, according to his peers.

For a man who likes being in clubs and societies, representing something is important. Arne is now Sweden's natural representative amongst the higher echelons of sport. However, it is not Arne who is important. The important thing is that Sweden as a nation is participating and making decisions, getting its voice heard. It is this that made it such an issue when there was no Swede who could succeed him when he left the IAAF. And there is a risk that the same thing may happen again with the IOC. The day that Arne steps down, he will not be succeeded by a Swede.

The International Olympic Committee has more than 110 members. It elects a president and an executive board who assemble in full approximately four times a year. The IOC assembles once a year in something that is called a 'session'. 'That's why the IOC is strongly led by its president. He has a large staff of employees who also have considerable influence.'

There are more than 200 national Olympic committees, and if every country was represented on the IOC like Sweden, with three members each, the IOC would have at least 600 members. It wouldn't work.

Arne has two colleagues from Sweden on the IOC. Gunilla Lindberg, the general secretary of the Swedish Olympic committee since 1989 was elected to the IOC in 1996. In 2004, she became only the second woman ever to become an IOC vice-president, a post from which she stepped down in August 2008 in Beijing. Göran Petersson is member since 2009 in his capacity as President of the International Sailing Federation.'

There is a custom that says those countries who have organised an Olympic Games have the right to two members of the IOC. Sweden last arranged an Olympic Games in 1912. 'I replaced Matts Carlgren in 1994, and Gunilla replaced Gunnar Ericsson two years later. We were both selected by direct order of IOC president Juan Antonio Samaranch, having been recommended by our predecessors.

'The Swedish Olympic committee thus had nothing to do with our nominations. We were selected on the basis of a purely direct order. Göran Petersson is elected as representative of the International Federations and will have to step down in 2012 when he reaches the age limit.

'IOC members are now elected according to a clearer nomination process than under Samaranch's time, following an appraisal and recommendations from a nomination committee. And the composition of the IOC's membership is regularly reviewed, as a large part of the world is not represented on the IOC. No matter how it comes to look in the future, this clearly means there is a risk that Sweden could also lose its representatives on the IOC. If this happens then it will undermine the chances of Sweden influencing on the policy of world sport and getting to host an Olympic Games in the future. Perhaps a Swede could become an IOC member one day in his or her capacity as the president of an international federation or representative of the athletes?

'It may be obvious, but it is true that the more representatives a country has, the more influence it has.

'It was awful to see what happened when Sweden had a chance to stage the 2014 Winter Olympics but the government decided not to give the necessary financial guarantees.

'I stick to what I wrote at the time: it is a scandal and I felt embarrassed to sit as a Swede on the IOC and discover that a wealthy country like Sweden doesn't feel that it has the resources to organise a Winter Games when other less wealthy countries like Kazakhstan and Bulgaria do. Still, Sweden likes to take part and pull off medals when they're on offer. It's disgraceful. If you're part of an international society you have to accept the terms and conditions, and that means offering something again.

'When it comes to a Swedish Olympic bid, it all comes down to applying with the right project at the right time. The Swedish bid for the 2004 Summer Olympics was the wrong project at the wrong time. The bid for the 1994 Winter Olympics probably was the right project at the right time. It was something of a shock that we got beaten by Lillehammer. We were close, I know. I don't know why we didn't win the ballot. Östersund 2014 would have had a good chance. My friends at the IOC more than raised their eyebrows when Östersund dropped out. It created an enormous surprise and astonishment which didn't do Sweden credit.'

'THERE ARE MANY who regard the IOC as a peculiar, impenetrable organisation. Like a kind of a gentleman's club. But it is not. There are many ladies involved, even though I think that there could be more. Really, it's not surprising that the IOC is rather closed. Nobody ought to complain about that. There are quite a lot of politicians who complain about the lack of democracy and goodness knows what else at the IOC, but that is based on ignorance and envy.

'I think that politicians are frustrated because they can't really control the IOC. They experience it as troublesome because the IOC is a very strong international force. Just look at those people who are on the IOC, look at their qualifications. It would be pretty hard to find as qualified and experienced a group in any other international context. Within the IOC, you find the most qualified expert knowledge about sport and considerable knowledge about society.

'In addition, there have been the IOC presidents. Sigrid J Edström was a Swedish pioneer. He was born in November 1870, he died in March 1964. He came from the world of industry, from Swedish company ASEA, where he was in charge between 1903 and 1933.

'After that he was chairman of the board until 1949. During his time, he also managed to take part in building up both the Swedish Federation of Industries and the

International Chamber of Commerce. He was also a sportsman. He was a sprinter, running 150 metres in 16.4 seconds back in 1891. He was vice-chairman of the organising committee for the 1912 Stockholm Olympics, a member of the IOC from 1920 until 1952, and president of the IOC from 1946 to 1952.

'It was also Edström who took the initiative to found the IAAF. He was IAAF president from 1913 to 1946. At home in Sweden he was involved in founding both the Swedish Gymnastics Association and the National Federation of Sporting Associations (*Idrottsföreningarnas riksförbund*) in 1903 and which was later renamed the Swedish Sports Confederation.

'Edström was followed as IOC president by Avery Brundage, an American. He was born in 1887 and died in 1975. Brundage was first and foremost a leader of sport, but he did have a short career as an active sportsman behind him. Among other things he participated in the 1912 Stockholm Olympics. He became president of the IOC in 1952 and remained so until 1972. He had been a member since 1936. Brundage was one of the people who most vigorously defended the principal that Olympic sportsmen should be amateurs. He also did a lot of work for his own country, serving as chairman of the United States Olympic Committee from 1929 until 1953, and as chairman of the national athletics governing body, the Amateur Athletic Union, from 1928 to 1933 and again in 1935.

'After Brundage, the IOC's president was drawn from the nobility. In 1927, the Irishman, Michael Morris Killanin succeeded to the title of Baron Killanin of Galway. It was Lord Killanin who modernised the Olympic movement. He became president in 1972 and remained in the position until 1980, when the Spanish marquis, Juan Antonio Samaranch, took over.

'Samaranch had built a political career with the Falangist Party, the Fascist movement that supported General Franco and wanted to construct a dictator state that closely followed old Catholic traditions. Samaranch had been the Spanish Minister of Sport from 1966 until 1970, having excelled as a sports official. He was a member of the Spanish Olympic Committee from 1955. Ten years later he joined the IOC, serving as vice-president between 1974 and 1978, when he then was made Spain's ambassador to Moscow. In 1980, he became the first full-time president of the IOC, a post he held until 2001.

'In comparison with Brundage, Samaranch was pragmatic, prepared to professionalise Olympic sport. The first step was to invite tennis players to be involved. It was a signal that we were breaking with the old model and ceasing to pretend that the top Olympic sportsmen weren't practising professionals. Samaranch had nothing against this.

'But when the IAAF introduced prize money for international athletics in conjunction with the 1993 world championships in Stuttgart, Samaranch was very worried. He thought that the IOC might be forced to do the same. He didn't want prize money involved in the Olympic Games. It was a concern that he expressed privately to me. I visited him twice a year to talk face-to-face. He wanted to talk to someone from the world of international athletics confidentially, and even though he and Primo Nebiolo were close, I don't think they were genuinely friends.

'Anyway, Samaranch talked to me about his concerns, which I can really understand. I shared his scepticism towards prize money in world championships. I thought then and still think now that the title of "world champion" should be prize enough, especially as winning the world title increases your worth to sponsors, so that you can rake money in.

'After Samaranch, a Belgian sports official by the name of Jacques Rogge took over as IOC president. Rogge was born in 1942 and became a member of the IOC in 1991. He is a good friend and colleague of mine. He is a doctor, an orthopaedic surgeon.

'I think Rogge is an excellent IOC president. Dynamic, and with a good background. When he became president he was the right age, and he had the right image. He is not quite as visible as Samaranch, but it is a completely different era now. During Samaranch's time we had the massive boycotts, the China–Taiwan issue, South Africa, and other political issues that kept cropping up. It required diplomatic intuition. Nowadays it's calmer.

'The one remaining burning issue today is doping, and being a doctor, Rogge is suitably qualified to tackle that. At the same time, though, that area of responsibility has been taken over by WADA.'

IT IS EASY to understand why Sweden's representation on international sporting bodies is close to Arne's heart. Having served international sport for half his life, he is respected and highly esteemed for his work. But Arne is not the only Ljungqvist in the history of Swedish sport, which sometimes leads to misunderstandings.

The other Swedish sports official named Ljungqvist was Rolf Ljungqvist, known usually as 'Lammet', 'the lamb'. He, too, was a doctor, but he specialised in tendons and was the first associate professor in the field of sports medicine in Sweden.

He crossed paths with Arne on several occasions. The first time was when he, in his capacity as a doctor with the Swedish athletics team, congratulated Arne on his victory in the high jump during the Finnkampen, the dual meeting against Finland, in 1951.

He greeted him by introducing himself as: 'Ljungqvist.'
'Yes, that's me,' replied Arne.

Even today there are still many sports people who refer to Arne as 'Lammet', even though they worked in different fields. 'Certainly, I get mixed up with "Lammet". It's happened on many official occasions, and that's not good. I also have a specific example that was particularly unpleasant. Ricky Bruch, the international discus thrower in the 1970s, once got "Lammet" to prescribe testosterone for him. With the prescription in his hand, Ricky approached the media and it became a real scandal. It was during the time that I was president of the Swedish athletics association. It was left to me to take care of the matter.

'It was not that long ago that a book was published in Canada which was based on an interview with a French doctor who alleged that it was I who gave Bruch the prescription. They used this to cast uncertainty on the suspicious figures who sit and decide over the anti-doping work around the world today. The main point of the book was to scandalise me and so undermine WADA and all its work being done to combat doping internationally.'

Of course, Arne responded to the book's desperate claims. He informed the publisher of the mix-up that had occurred and the whole thing ended up with the authorities confiscating the entire print run of books. 'I met the author later at the Turin Olympic Games and said to him that it would perhaps have been better if he had called the person he was accusing and double-checked if it was true. I could see he was embarrassed.'

When Rolf "Lammet" Ljungqvist died in 1990, it was Arne who gave a speech for his namesake at the funeral which took place at Gustav Vasa Church in Stockholm.

Chapter 15

Celebrities and Money

THE INTERNATIONAL OLYMPIC Committee. The International Association of Athletics Federations. The World Anti-Doping Agency. Arne's involvement has taken him into the inner circles of world sport. It has given him the influence and the power to shape and change opinions about doping and other medically related matters and achieve success in tackling them.

It has also given him prestige. Without really knowing how, he has become famous. He moves like a fish in water alongside other sporting celebrities. Many Olympic and world championship heroes have, after retiring from competing, continued to represent their country as sports officials and they now attend the same meetings as Arne.

'Being a celebrity has meant that people want me to attend all sorts of events, one strange one after another. At one time I was invited to all kinds of galas, parties and openings, but I have consistently declined if it hasn't had anything to do with what I was committed to doing. I have never been interested in that kind of life. I'm instinctively sceptical of celebrity.'

One thing his involvement in international sport has not given Arne is a massive income. His work for sport has been voluntary. There has been no difference between working for Bromma IF, the local athletics club he helped set up in the suburbs of Stockholm when he was a youngster, and the IOC. 'When I think that I have worked my entire life as a sports official without pay, it feels pretty good. Leading a voluntary organisation has the benefit of working without your self-interest at heart. You don't have those kind of loyalties. Besides, it's the employees who carry out the work. They're the ones who should be well-paid.

'I'm thinking about when we started Bromma IF. There were two people who helped us get the club up and running. Those two people, and the volunteering leaders from the time I was an athlete, are my role models. They personify for me the idealistic leadership which is the great strength of Swedish sport. Unfortunately there is a growing notion gaining support, even in Sweden, that officials who lead sport should be paid. For my part, I am glad that I worked voluntarily and without pay, but I think it will be difficult to maintain that kind of tradition in the future.'

Arne was not without offers from industry. 'But I've consistently declined. I haven't wanted to be involved in trade and industry; instead, I've tried to keep away from all kinds of work which would be incompatible with my independence, even though it might be lucrative. In the same way I've always stepped down from projects which could come into conflict with any new undertakings that I've made.

'For example, I stepped down from the IAAF's medical committee, which I'd chaired for twenty years, when I was asked to take over the chairmanship of the IOC's medical commission. I wanted to avoid any risk of being accused of favouring athletics within the IOC.'

Arne has always been very careful to control his public life. Just as he has tried to keep a distinction between his private life and professional work, he has also strictly kept himself to only those arenas connected with his experience and professional competence. But his commitment and involvement has also earned him considerable respect, not just from colleagues within the world of sport or competing athletes.

Having worked voluntarily for so many years, though, has had some economic benefits. 'I attended a WADA meeting in Tallinn in 2001, and when I went down to check out of the hotel, I saw Anders Flodström had called. He was then the vice-chancellor of the Royal Institute of Technology (KTH).

'Because we are on the board of the same research grant committee, I thought it must have something to do with that. I called him up immediately and asked what the matter was.

'"It's about you, Arne," he said. "You've been awarded the Royal Institute of Technology's most senior prize – for the work you've done to combat doping. For the success you have had with your research background. For the important work you've done for young people in Sweden and internationally. And the prize isn't just an honour: you'll receive a tiny sum of money too."

'I was pleasantly surprised. My first thought was that perhaps I could take Ulla out to dinner. "Yes," continued Flodström, "it's 900,000 kronor tax-free."'

The prize is about the same as US$140,000. 'My God,' I thought. 'Tax-free!'

The prize was provided by an anonymous benefactor some time in the 1940s when a huge amount of money was donated. In the letter that accompanied the donation, he or she stipulated that the recipient of the award would be free to use the money as he or she saw fit, without having to account for it. The prize is incredibly prestigious, both in Sweden and outside the country. 'And I knew that. I'm a member of the Royal *Medaljnämnd* – the Swedish honours committee. I know what the Swedish honours systems looks like. I didn't know that KTH-prize was so much money, though.'

The prize was awarded during a ceremony and banquet in the Golden Hall at Stockholm City Hall on November 16, 2001.

THE WORLD OF SPORT is full of colourful personalities. If you spend your whole life there, as Arne has done, you have many memories, of people you've met, admired or worked with.

One of the first in a long line is a Swedish namesake, Arne Borg. Borg was one of the top international swimmers in the 1920s and one of the first major sporting icons. He won four Olympic medals, set thirty-two world records and won forty Swedish championships.

'You wouldn't have put money on me meeting him because he had retired before I was even born. I remember that my mother and father met him once at a mutual friend's party. I must have been eight or ten at the time. My mother said that he had been so "full of fun".

'Borg eventually died in 1987, but just a short time before that I gave him a lift home from a meeting at the head office of a sports federation. It was then that I understood what my mother had meant.

'Borg had a colossal gallows humour, and I took the scenic route to his home north of Stockholm as much as I dared just to be able to listen to him for as long as possible. When we parted, he said that he thought it was fun meeting me. But it was even funnier for me.'

Another namesake that Arne got to meet was Arne Andersson, the middle-distance runner, who together with Gunder Hägg broke so many world records.

Andersson was born in 1917 and died in 2009. He set four world records during his career. He was banned for breaking the amateur rules in 1946, along with Hägg. 'As a child I had seen both Arne and Gunder and I could well comprehend the adult feeling of catastrophe when the two of them were told they would never get to race again.

'Many years later, I got to telephone Arne Andersson to tell him that we at the IAAF had lifted his ban. Arne Andersson was very touched when he understood why I contacted him. We had arranged for a journalist from *Göteborgs-Posten* to be at Arne's home when I called, so that the paper could take pictures when he got my message. He was so incredibly happy. It was important for him.

'Gunder Hägg, on the other hand, didn't care. "Once a professional – always a professional," was his sole comment.'

There are other examples, of foreign athletes who have won the favour of the Swedish public and almost been adopted by the nation, whom Arne got to meet. One of them is Emil Zatopek, from Czechoslovakia, one of the greatest long-distance runners of all time. During his career he won 261 of the 334 races in which he competed. In eighteen of them, he set a world record. He is still today the only athlete who has ever won the 5000 metres, 10,000 metres and the marathon during the same Olympics.

'It was at the same Olympics that I got to participate in as a high jumper in Helsinki in 1952. I got to know him later in his life. We met occasionally in different VIP boxes during the 1990s when he came to look at athletics events.

I admired him not just for his sporting achievements but also because he was so fearless. After he had already retired from sport, during the "Prague Spring' uprising of 1968, he took part and signed a petition demanding democracy. As punishment, he was demoted and kicked out of the defence ministry where he worked. Until then, he had been a colonel in the army. He was thrown out of the Czech Communist party and all his allowances and benefits were immediately withdrawn.

'It was only after democracy came to Czechoslovakia in 1990 that he was reinstated as a colonel.'

The history of sport is closely entwined with political events. 'One athlete who I really admired from childhood was the Korean runner, the marathon winner in Berlin in 1936, Kee-Chung Sohn.

'Because Korea was occupied by Japan at that time, he was forced to run for Japan. It was not until after the war, at the Olympics in London in 1948, that Sohn was able to run for his native South Korea. And at the 1988 Seoul Olympics, it was Sohn who carried the Olympic flame into the stadium, which was an enormous occasion, especially for the Korean nation.

'I met him in South Korea on a few occasions and I gathered that he was bitter that he had been forced to win the medal for Japan. And even if I never really got to know him because of the language barrier, it was undeniably wonderful to get to shake hands with him and sit down and, with the help of an interpreter, talk to him.'

Arne has had lots of conversations like that over the years. It has been everything from politely curious conversations in the stands overlooking a track somewhere in the world, to deeper discussions at meetings of different international sporting organisations. Some of them have developed over the years and grown into firm friendships.

'It was particularly special, of course, to meet Dick Fosbury and hear the story about the flop technique direct from the man that invented it. He revolutionised the high jump, but if you look back at recordings from 1968, you see how undeveloped the technique was. Fosbury lies with his back almost completely flat over the bar. He gains height by lifting his bottom.

'Stefan Holm's modern technique is much more advanced. He arcs his back over the bar and gains even more height in doing so.

'The Soviet high jumper Valeriy Brumel used a completely different technique. He had a fantastic straddle style. Meeting him was a lot of fun. It was actually Brumel who looked *me* up. He wanted to give me a wristwatch in honour of what I had done for sport and because I was an old high jumper. I still have it. Brumel's career was cut short when he was just twenty-three, after a motorcycle accident. As I had also been forced to retire after my knee injury early in my career, I knew fully well what he felt. We talked about it when we met.'

FOSBURY IS AMONG a special category of athletes who revolutionised their event. They 'chiselled out something new,' as Arne says. 'Another example is Jan Boklöv, who revolutionised ski jumping. He used a style we call the "V-technique" in Sweden but which was initially known as the Boklöv-technique by the rest of the world. Isn't it typically Swedish that we can't even honour our own sportsmen and women better?'

The naturally athletically talented also deserve mention. Carl Lewis belongs to that group. 'I've already talked about him. Jesse Owens also belongs to that group of special athletes. In 1935, Owens jumped 8.16 metres in the long jump, on a cinder track and off a wooden take-off board;

he did the 200 metres in 20.2 and the 100 metres in 10.2 seconds. All this was more than seventy-five years ago on the running tracks of his day.

'A third figure was decathlete Bob Mathias, who was just seventeen years old and had only been training a few months when he broke through and won the decathlon at the 1948 London Olympics. He then successfully defended his title at the 1952 Helsinki Olympics.

'There are many others, such as the Brazilian footballer Pelé, whom I met when he visited the Beijing Games.

'And there was the discus thrower Al Oerter, who won gold at every Olympics from 1956 to 1968 and had extraordinary technique.

'One athlete who never received this kind of celebrity attention but who was far ahead of his time was the pole vaulter, Cornelius Warmerdam, who set three world records between 1940 and 1942. The highest was 4.77 metres, with a bamboo pole, a record that remained in place until 1957 when a new type of aluminum pole had been developed. To jump so high on a cinder track with a rigid stick is quite amazing.'

Among the foremost talents there are also tragic examples of careers that were cut short, through accidents, like Brumel's, or bans, like Hägg and Andersson. 'Jim Thorpe, who competed in the pentathlon and decathlon, is another example. At the 1912 Stockholm Olympics these were new events and Jim Thorpe won both the pentathlon and decathlon hands down. He received a cup from King Gustaf V and the Russian Tsar Nikolai II.

'Famously, at the prize-giving ceremony, the Swedish king said: "You are the greatest athlete in the world", to which Thorpe replied, "Thanks King."

'But Thorpe was stripped of his medals the following year for breaking the amateur rules. He had played baseball the year before the Games and received fifteen dollars a week. The rules were rock solid in those days. So Thorpe carried on with baseball, and he also got involved in an undistinguished acting career. But he was already an alcoholic which, in 1953, cost him his life.

'In 1983, the IOC decided to return the medals to his family, following which a memorial ceremony took place in the Stockholm Olympic Stadium.'

THE HISTORY OF sport is full of unforgettable moments, of victories and defeats. Arne has found himself in both situations. Both when competing in the arena and when watching from the sidelines.

'I remember the time in Stockholm in 1940 when Gunder Hägg broke through, on the heels of Henry Kälarne when he set a world record in the 3,000 metres. There shouldn't have been anyone close to him. Kälarne was the bronze medallist from the 5000 metres at the 1936 Berlin Olympics.

'Yet along comes a totally unknown lad, almost catching up with him. In terms of the emotion, for me that moment only compares to the time when I, as a twelve-year-old, won all the events at my school championships in 1943, or when I, six years later, won three of the four events to win the Kunngakann Trophy for Bromma Secondary School. And, of course, when I made my debut for the Swedish national team in the 1951 Finnkampen. Those are four moments in my early sporting days that I look back upon.'

But Arne remembers to point out that the history of sport also contains tragedies of a completely different kind. 'I was at the 1972 Munich Olympic Games. Matts Carlgren had taken me there to look and learn, and as the hotel I was staying at was right next to the

Olympic Village, I found myself close to the site of the massacre.

'My room was on the third floor, overlooking the grass court where the helicopters landed to take the terrorists away with their hostages. So when the hostages were loaded into helicopters and flown away, I stood watching. I did not dare have the light on in my room, and while I watched, I listened to the news on the radio. They said that a raid had taken place, the terrorists had been killed and the hostages had been freed. Tragically, that was far from the truth.

'The attack had taken place at night, and those of us who were left at the hotel found out what had happened. But Matts had already gone sight-seeing with the rest of the Swedish athletics team. So he didn't know what had happened. That day was free from athletics competitions and when Matts got back, reporters from Swedish national television were waiting for him by the barriers. He was asked if he had any comment to make on what had happened during the day.

'Not knowing what was going on, he started talking about how the Swedish team was feeling, a few injuries and so on. When they broadcast the news item about the terrorist attack they edited in Matts' comments, which looked really ridiculous given what had happened. Matts was extremely disappointed. Personally, I learned to be very careful giving taped interviews and always find out when and how it's to be broadcast.'

FOUR NAMES FROM modern Swedish athletics have a particular significance for Arne. They are Anders Gärderud, the steeplechaser who won gold at the 1976 Montreal Olympics, during Arne's time as president of Swedish athletics. Then there is Patrik Sjöberg, the high jumper who set a world record at Stockholm Stadium in 1987: Arne's old event at Arne's own arena.

The third is Stefan Holm, who in dramatic circumstances in 2004, won what was up to that point Sweden's only Olympic gold medal for the high jump.

The fourth is Ludmila Engqvist, the hurdler who won gold at the 1996 Atlanta Olympics. She became a favourite in Sweden but was subsequently caught doping. For the second time.

So why has Arne chosen Ludmila?

'Because she came back in 1999 after suffering cancer. She was cleared of the first doping charges in 1995 but that the whole thing took a tragic turn when she was caught doping in 2001 is another story. It can't detract from the enormous fight she made with herself and her bitter fate. That she was diagnosed with cancer having just turned thirty, went through treatment with an operation and chemotherapy, and then made her comeback. It wasn't thanks to doping that she was able to make a comeback. She was under incredible medical scrutiny. I know that because I helped her get treatment.

'When the cancer was discovered, Ludmila and her husband Johan contacted me, writing me a letter in their panic. I don't think it's an exaggeration to put it like that. They were in Spain and didn't know what to do, how to get help and what help might be available in Sweden.

'I followed her illness closely until her treatment was over. I know what pain she went through, and what personal strength she had. When she made her comeback at the DN-Gala in Stockholm while still going through chemotherapy I couldn't believe my eyes.

'It is incomprehensible how Ludmila and Johan could later take a gamble by her doping. She had taken pills to help her put on weight ahead of her attempt to do bobsleigh. The first thing they did when they realised what the situation was regarding her doping test was to call me. They wanted to tell me personally before news got out. I would be very disappointed, they said, and they knew that they had let me down and all that ... and that was that. After the second doping scandal I haven't had much contact with either Ludmila or Johan, but they get in touch by text message occasionally. The fact that they let me down does not take anything away from the greatness Ludmila showed during her illness.'

The phenomenon that was Ludmila Engquist is a reminder about another thing. Sweden is a small country, one that has not had much experience of having much immigration. So it has not had experience of producing a national team with great ethnic variety, unlike some other European nations.

'At the 1996 Olympics in Atlanta, Ludmila won gold for Sweden. When a nation wins gold, it is common for the heads of the other national teams to congratulate the head of the winning team. So it was now. But the leaders of the Swedish team started to dismiss her achievement, because she was "really" Russian. Certainly, she'd run in Swedish colours, but she was a Russian.

'The heads of the other international teams just didn't get it. A French team manager said: "Good lord, half our team comes from other parts of the world." It gave all our team leaders, and not just me, something to think about. We should be happy that boys and girls become Swedes and represent our country in a good way.

'But this can also be a complicated issue. There are countries nowadays that recruit elite sportsmen and women by offering them citizenship and other benefits, which I think is wrong. It is a problem we're trying to combat right now within international sport. How can we establish rules and regulations for which country an athlete can represent without it coming into conflict with other national and international laws?'

Chapter 16

Ulla and Shared Memories

ULLA HAS BEEN the joy of Arne's life. The first time they saw each other she was thirteen. Arne was fifteen. They were at school. The year was 1946.

Her father had a boat down near Ålsten's harbour. Arne's mate had one down there too. And during the summer of 1947, Ulla and Arne's paths crossed again and again. When autumn came, it was time for the school dances.

At least once a month, there was a dance. It was a focal point where all the friends could meet. Then there were also film shows on Monday evenings. They hired in cinema films and showed them on an old projector in the school hall, with the film interrupted every time they had to change the reel.

It was at one of those film evenings one autumn, when the reel was being changed and the light in the school hall was on, that Arne saw Ulla again. 'She was so incredibly sweet, and she stood up and looked around as if she wanted to be noticed.'

At the next school dance, Arne invited Ulla to dance. It was October 7, 1947.

After that, they met often and, eventually, Arne was invited to Ulla's home, and from that day on they considered themselves a couple. 'Ulla and I were together a lot that first year. I must admit that it was so intense that Ulla's schoolwork suffered and she had to repeat a year. Her father viewed it very seriously, but her mother was a bit more understanding.'

Her parents weren't like others at that time. Both were employed. It was unusual for a mother to have a job if she had two children of school age. Ulla's mother worked full-time at the central post office on Vasagatan in central Stockholm, which she loved. Her father also worked for the post office and eventually went on to become one of the directors there. Ulla grew up in a house, just like Arne, not far from the sports ground at Stora Mossen.

On winter evenings in the living room you could hear music from the ice rink in the stadium where people got together to skate. But the family would soon move into an apartment in newly built Abrahamsberg because, as both parents were working, they didn't have time to look after a big house and garden. Now they were near to the trams and buses, to the services of the day, in a nice, clean newly built area.

Arne often visited Ulla after they started dating. He was well liked and her parents got involved in the young couple's relationship is an unusually trusting way. 'One time Ulla and I had been quarrelling – this must have been something like 1949 or 1950 – and Ulla had run home to her mother and complained or said something and started crying. So Ulla's mother picked up the phone and called me and told me that Ulla was confused and wanted to know how things stood between us. It shows what kind of relationship we had: that Ulla's mother felt able to talk to me about the problem in that way. I said what I thought, that it was a bit of a falling out and that I knew that I wanted to be with Ulla.'

Arne and Ulla dated for a long time before they even thought about getting engaged. But that day came on June 5, 1954. They had picked out a romantic spot for the event together, a rock in Solvikskogen forest in Ålsten. From the rock they had a wonderful view over Lake Mälaren. 'Afterwards we had an engagement dinner at Stallmästaregården – a fine restaurant in Stockholm. We had chicken. This was party food at that time. It was early summer and I remember that Ulla didn't feel very well. She kept thinking about her mother's illness.'

Just before their engagement, Ulla's mother had become very sick and she hadn't been able to work. She told Ulla that it was serious. An infection had caused her kidneys to shrivel up. She was only fifty-five years old. Ulla became incredibly sad. She was very close to her mother. 'I can't help but think that if she had got the disease just ten to fifteen years later, it would have been possible to save her life through a transplant. But back then they didn't do such operations.'

Ulla's mother was in and out of hospital over a long period. People with chronic kidney disease often develop anaemia. Frequent blood transfusions were necessary. Nowadays such anaemia is treated with erythropoietin (EPO), which increases the number of red blood cells. EPO, of course, has also been used in sports doping.

When Ulla's mother got sick, medical science didn't know why poorly functioning kidneys led to anaemia. We know now that it is in the kidneys that the human body produces EPO. When the kidneys cease to function, the body stops producing EPO.

Ulla's mother died in 1959. Her father didn't reach old age either. He was just sixty-three years old, in the autumn of 1963, when he was hit by a cancer that would take his life within six months.

Ulla graduated from high school in 1953 with such good grades that she got into *Gymnastiska centralinstitutet*. She studied to be a physiotherapist, and she graduated in 1956. The same summer Arne completed enough of his medical studies that he was able to work as a temporary assistant physician. That autumn Ulla and Arne moved to north Sweden, where they both got temporary positions at various hospitals. It was somewhere up north that they decided that it was time to get married, and it was also somewhere up north where Mats was conceived, because when they got married at Bromma Church on March 23, 1957, Ulla was already pregnant.

Bromma's is one of the oldest churches in Sweden. It is not particularly big, but splendid as it is situated not far from the lake Bromma Kyrksjö. Both Ulla and Arne were popular with lots of friends, and both families were close knit; Arne's sporting friends also came, even though his active days as an athlete were over. So it was in front of a packed congregation that Ulla and Arne tied the knot, the service taken by the vicar who had confirmed them both in their teens.

AFTER THEY WERE married, Arne and Ulla moved in together. They lived for a short time in a newly built two-room apartment in Fruängen, in the south of Stockholm. But the whole street at Fruängsgatan was like a building site and they yearned for their old suburb.

As soon as a larger apartment became available in a part of Bromma named Råcksta, they moved there. Arne finished his medical studies and started off working as a locum doctor, but as soon as he got his post at the department of pathology at the Karolinska Institutet, the Ljungqvist family had a modest but steady income. Mats was small and Ulla stayed home. She soon got pregnant again. In 1960, Håkan was born.

It was about this time that many young families bought their own homes and Arne and Ulla were no different. They got the idea of owning a home from their parents. 'When I got a permanent job at the department of pathology, I wasn't really rich, but at least I had a steady income. I was working on a research project with a friend at the radiological department, and one day he told me that I ought to think about my living situation and perhaps think about buying my own home. "You're crazy," I told him. "I can't afford that."

'But he had just bought a house and was really satisfied with it. I didn't know very much about personal finances so I rang up my parents and some relatives. They offered to lend me the money.'

Ulla and Arne caught sight of a house in Enebyberg in the township of Danderyd north of Stockholm. It was a long way from the city. It was like moving out to the country, but a second-hand car could get them to and from work and the shops. Danderyd was a market town at that time, picturesque and tranquil. The house they wanted was for sale because the owner wanted an apartment in Stockholm.

'He'd built the house himself and lived there for fifteen years. The best thing about it was that the house was built in agreement with the local municipality. In those days, to encourage people to move there, if you built and lived in your own house in a market town, you got a good loan and the land for half the price. We got to take over a really good value loan.'

In 1962, Arne and Ulla's growing family moved out to the house in Enebyberg. Maria, Ulla's and Arne's third child, was born in 1964. Arne still lives there to this day.

AS THE YEARS passed, soon even Maria had grown up and started school. Ulla and Arne agreed that Ulla shouldn't stay home anymore, but she was worried that her education wouldn't suffice after all the years she had been a housewife. 'She didn't know if she dared take up a career again. But there was a refresher course for physiotherapists. It was set up for one reason: most physiotherapists were women and so many of them became housewives that the care industry needed to get them back as staff. But Ulla said that she didn't want to. She was scared. She wouldn't be able to manage. Not even the course.

'So I signed her up on my own initiative for the refresher course at Karolinska University Hospital (KS). It was 1971 she got this as her birthday present. "Now you're signed up!" I told her, and she was upset and happy all at once. When she finally did the refresher course, it went really well. She got really good evaluations and the patients loved her. Straight after the course she was hired at KS.'

Arne had had his post at KS for a while. Now they could travel to work together. Ulla chose to work part-time, so she could still be responsible for the home and children. That was how she wanted it.

One of the senior physiotherapists at KS was Mari-Ann Frösell who, when she decided to open a private practice at her home in Djursholm, asked Ulla if she would like to join the new company. 'It was incredibly flattering for Ulla. Mari-Ann was one of the stars at KS. And Djursholm was not far from Enebyberg. Ulla jumped at the chance, happy that she only worked part-time at KS. Now she could work the other fifty per cent of her time with Mari-

Ann. When she got fed up working in two different places, she quit working in the city and started working full-time at Mari-Ann's.'

Ulla and Mari-Ann worked together throughout the 1980s, but when Mari-Ann became very ill and died in the early 1990s, Ulla was left alone with the business. 'At the same time I was getting many major assignments that required me to travel all over the world.' The year was 1993. The children had all left home, and Ulla chose to end her working career, retiring aged sixty. Arne thought it was a good decision. Now he and Ulla could be together on the trips. Ulla could come with him as a representative and see the world.

TO BEGIN WITH, they had a great time together with their new life. But their future wasn't to be as they had imagined. They weren't to grow old in comfort together. Ulla developed Alzheimer's. Maybe she even had the first signs when she retired. The illness was to turn their last years together into a nightmare.

'I don't really know exactly when it started. I ought to have noticed. But you don't. Alzheimer's is an incredibly insidious illness. When you live so closely intertwined, as Ulla and I did, the first signs pass you by. You've grown so much together that you don't notice the small changes. But it was at some point towards the middle of the 1990s that her memory began to fail. I don't know if there was any connection, but about the time when the Estonia ferry sank in the autumn of 1994, Ulla went into a deep depression. I don't think it had anything to do with the deaths of all those people, but both events are in some way connected in my mind.

'Ulla was so bad that I contacted a psychiatrist. It's not uncommon that depression comes in the first stages of Alzheimer's. It could be the case that the depression was set off because Ulla herself noticed that she wasn't functioning well.'

Ulla received treatment and slowly fought her way up out of depression. When she was better, Arne didn't think any more about it. Life was back to normal. Ulla was able to undergo a successful hip operation, and was really happy with the outcome. 'But a year later she started getting a lot of bad pain in her operated hip. The doctors couldn't find out what was causing the pain. I assumed that it was just muscle contraction that a good physiotherapist would be able to alleviate, but her doctor thought otherwise and was of the opinion that the muscle was inflamed.

'Ulla was given Voltaren for the pain, a non-steroid anti-inflammatory medicine that is often given to athletes. Then, one day, Ulla had acute heart failure. It's known that Voltaren can damage the heart, so she was taken into KS.'

A friend of Arne's, Bosse Berglund, a doctor at KS and chief medical officer for the Olympic team, saw Ulla when she was admitted. He was of the opinion that Ulla was very overweight because of too much fluid in her body. It wasn't difficult to reduce the fluid and give her restorative heart medicine. But Bosse also noted that Ulla couldn't account for herself or explain what had happened. And that was something he wanted explained so he admitted Ulla for two days. It was 1999.

'Bosse told me about what he had observed. From that day on I tried to persuade Ulla to undergo a memory test. There are memory clinics after all, and at Huddinge University Hospital there's a "Memory Centre" which Bosse suggested, either there or at Danderyd hospital where they are really good. But Ulla flew into a rage every time I tried to bring the matter up.

'It's clear she had an idea of what was happening, but she pretended she didn't. She didn't want to hear any mention of it and every time I said something, it felt like I was trampling all over something that was incredibly private. This was how it carried on: I persisted; she was angry; and so the years passed. But I had started to notice things and saw that it wasn't working. Everyday life became more and more problematic and when travelling abroad, I had to keep more and more of an eye on her. In the end I wouldn't even let her go into the city on her own because I didn't know what would happen. Each time she took the car to nearby Täby Centrum for shopping I had butterflies in my stomach. She started asking about the same things, small things which I knew she knew and I noticed that I was getting more and more irritated with her. It became imperative for her to be examined.'

Arne contacted Bosse Berglund again. Almost four years had passed since Ulla had been admitted for heart failure. Her hip pain was long since gone and her heart medication was efficient. She was in physically good condition. Bosse wrote a referral and Ulla was called in for a memory examination by the care centre. When they rang, Ulla answered. 'She didn't understand what it was about. So I lied and told her it was her cardiologist who wanted to see if her medication had any side-effects. It was what I blamed it on just to get things going again. I was forced to.'

A comprehensive testing on Ulla's memory started in 2003. They did isotope studies of the brain, a brain scan and lumbar punctures, at the same time as other tests and discussions. Testing still wasn't complete by summer of 2004, and Arne and Ulla travelled together to the Olympics in Athens. When they got back, Ulla's diagnosis was ready.

'All the tests had been analysed and we were called in to the geriatric clinic at Danderyd. I don't know how many times I've been present to give a patient a diagnosis, often a terminal one. But now we were sitting on the other side of the table, waiting for Ulla's diagnosis. It was Alzheimer's. I don't think Ulla understood what was said. It's possible the illness had already gone too far or she just blocked it out. I don't know.'

ARNE IS NOW alone with his memories of Ulla. Of their life together and the years with the illness. Where did it start? When did it take his Ulla from him? He remembers an incident in the spring of 2003. Ulla had received the appointment to go and undergo tests on memory and they had gone out to the island of Blidö, to their summer house, and sat together in the sunshine and talked. 'She suddenly got really confused while we were sitting there. She started crying and said: "I'm ruining it for you."' Perhaps on some level Ulla understood what was happening to her. Even if it was for just an instant.

'When we arrived at the clinic for the test on that very first day, I was genuinely scared. The doctor asked what year it was, and Ulla answered: "Well, yes it's 2000 ... and something." It really was that bad! Later, she had to draw a geometric figure but she couldn't get the lines to go together in the pentagon or whatever it was. She couldn't join the lines up.'

Arne has searched his memory to try to remember the first signs of Ulla's illness. But it is impossible to say when it all began. As early as six years or more before the diagnosis there were times when Ulla was disorientated or forgot what she had to do. Was that the illness? Was that the first sign? Often, she went her own way, reacting irrationally in what had previously been familiar situations. 'It occurs to me that Ulla had stopped reading books around 2000, even though she had been a real bookworm before, devouring stacks of books. I remember that she commented on it herself. "It's weird," she said. "I don't read books anymore."'

Great sporting events provide a reliable calendar to key memories. Each occasion belongs to an event and a year, and each year there is trip to a championships or an Olympics.

'In 2001 the IAAF world championships were held in Edmonton, Canada. I remember that we were at an outdoor museum when I stopped to talk with a few friends and got a bit separated from the others. Ulla was so angry. She really lost her temper and thought that I had left her. It was completely bizarre, but I understood even then what was behind it. The interesting thing was that our Chinese friends, Lou Dapeng and his family (Lou was then one of the vice-presidents of the IAAF) had noticed that there was something wrong with Ulla. Mrs Lou and Ulla were the best of friends, and when on some other occasion they were to take part in some social activity or another while we men were at a meeting, she said to me in her polite, reserved manner: "Don't worry, Arne. I'll take care of Ulla."'

The following year, Arne and Ulla were in Montreal. Arne had a meeting with WADA during the day and they were going to meet up again at the hotel at 7p.m. to get ready for the official dinner. Ulla had accompanied Arne on hundreds of official occasions like this, she was always sure of herself, happy, appreciated and well-liked by people.

'When I got back to our hotel room at 7p.m., Ulla wasn't there. I was forced to ring the organiser and say that we couldn't come to the dinner because Ulla had vanished.

Not even my closest colleagues knew about her illness. I couldn't keep it from them any more. Quickly, I informed them. It was then eight o'clock. The hotel security had been notified and in turn they contacted the police, who checked the hospitals. They told me not to worry and that they were sure they would find Ulla. "She's somewhere in town," they said. "If something had happened to her we would know about it."

'Two hours later reception called. Ulla had returned. She had been in the shopping mall just opposite the hotel. She was happy and beaming, greeted the policeman and asked what they were doing there. She didn't have a clue what was going on. "My dear," I said. "We should have been at the dinner several hours ago."

'"I didn't know that," she answered. "You didn't say anything about it."

'During the world championships in Paris in 2003, there were no major incidents. It also went well in Athens in 2004, but I had to write notes to Ulla with times and where she could get hold of me.' Arne didn't dare leave Ulla alone after what happened in Montreal. On trips when Arne was going to spend most of his time at different meetings, she was no longer able to come. Arne began to take a detour to Luxembourg, where their son Mats lived and worked, so Ulla could stay there while he was away.

The following year, 2005, it was the world championships in Helsinki. As usual, Arne was present as an official. Ulla had always accompanied him. Over the years she had built up her own social network within the society of sport. This time was different. Arne travelled over to Helsinki on his own to take part in the IAAF congress and council meeting. Ulla stayed behind on the island of Blidö in the Stockholm archipelago together with the children, who also spend their summer there. She felt at home on Bildö, having first gone there as a small child. After a few days, Arne returned to collect Ulla and take her to Helsinki. 'I thought we should be together and see the championships. Ulla was delighted. But then one morning when there were no events, the council wanted to have a short meeting. I explained to Ulla that I would only be away for a short while and that she should stay in the hotel room while I was away. She didn't need to worry. The meeting was to be held in a drawing room at the hotel and I wouldn't be gone very long.

'In the middle of the meeting, someone rushed in saying that Ulla was wandering around the corridors, disorientated. She didn't know which room she was staying in. I left the meeting but Ulla had already vanished from the hotel. They soon found her. Ulla was well-known and liked to talk to people. It turned out that there was a chap there at the hotel who was on his way to the stadium to do something. Ulla had asked if she could go with him. The arena was deserted except for Ulla, who sat there completely alone in the VIP stand. It was dreadful. It's a horrendous illness. And with her illness, she went into rapid decline.'

ULLA BEGAN TO take medication for her illness in the autumn of 2004. She was given a cholinesterase-inhibitor, but it is hard to know if it helped. Slowly, she became increasingly confused. Sometimes, she didn't even recognise Arne. Home wasn't home any more. She was always packing to go home to her mother in Bromma. She began to see people that weren't there. There were people who were going to throw them out of the house in Enebyberg, because it wasn't theirs. She confused the house on Blidö with the one her parents once had on the island. 'She asked me what her father would say about the new house – our summer house. I tried to explain to her that her father had been dead for more than forty years, but no, that wasn't so. And the most frightening thing about this was that Ulla saw me as mad. What she experienced was real to her.'

Arne realised that it couldn't go on. Ulla needed full-time care. He contacted the local healthcare authority who organised temporary care for her in sheltered accommodation. 'Each time I went away, I could leave her there. There was no way she could live on her own any more.'

In January 2006, Arne made one last desperate attempt to take Ulla to Mats in Luxembourg while he went to a WADA meeting in Montreal. But Arne had barely arrived in Montreal when Mats called. 'He was desperately upset. "Mamma's mad," he said. "She doesn't know where she is and she doesn't recognise me. She's aggressive and is packing her bags and going home." I sat there in Canada and could only say to Mats to try and get her to take the medicine I had left him. It lessened her anxiety. He finally sorted it. Perhaps it was good that even Mats got to see what was happening to his mother.

'When I left her with Mats in Luxembourg, I had had to coax her and tell her that she would be much better there and that I was just going to be at meetings the whole time. After what happened though, it wasn't possible to leave her with Mats any more so I had to use the temporary care instead.

'Each time I had to pretend and say that she was just going there for a short visit. When I later picked her up, she didn't know if she had been there for a day or a week. She was so bad then. It's almost impossible to describe how it is to live with a person who is suffering from Alzheimer's.'

Even so, Arne told their mutual friends in the world of sport about Ulla's illness early on. Eventually he told the press and he allowed the evening tabloids to tell his and Ulla's story. 'I made a choice to be open about what was happening to the family and the tragedy that had struck Ulla. There's no reason to hide it. Both because it's impossible to do that and because it's a relief to be able to share something so awful with other people.'

Ulla's illness continued to worsen. She forgot where things were kept. She couldn't use the coffee maker. She couldn't tell the difference between the washing machine and the dryer. She didn't understand why everything went wrong, and this in turn made her angry. She began to scream and argue.

'Our existence became incredibly chaotic. It's awful to stand there and watch it happen to your partner. Ulla and I had lived together for such a long time that we had become one. It's like a part of me has faded and gone.

'At times we were sitting there talking and she would suddenly turn to me and ask: "Who are you?" And when I, surprised, would tell her that I was Arne, that we had lived our lives together and loved each other since we were at school, she would sarcastically laugh right in my face and say: "You're mad!"

'"Who am I then?" I would ask Ulla. "I've no idea," she would reply. "But what am I doing here then?" I would ask. "It's good you're here," she would tell me.

'There were times when Ulla became violent and attacked me. When I wasn't looking she would hide the post. And then at other times she could come to me when I was sitting at the computer and say: "I wonder when Arne is coming?"

'What the hell! It's just not possible to live in such an absurd daily life. The worst thing was that you had to keep yourself together all the time, be understanding and not get cross because that only made things worse.'

Ulla became completely uninterested in her children and grandchildren. She barely knew they existed. Sometimes she could improve a little when they came, but it quickly passed. 'In the winter of 2006, she packed her bags practically every day and was going to leave but I managed to keep her home. It was an awful time. One day I heard her packing really thoroughly. Then she went down the stairs to go out. She had found her outdoor clothes but had no idea that there was a snowstorm outside. "Well, I'm going home," she said. That's how it was again and again. Again I had to explain that she was already home. "Please Ulla, you can't go now." I looked in the plastic bag that she was standing there holding, "What have you got there?" And I saw that she had packed an apron and a pair of shoes. And now she was ready to go home with that baggage after hours of packing. I could have cried. So I opened the door and we could see it was a snowstorm. "You can't go now in this weather," I said. Then she went inside again. It was awful.'

IN MARCH 2006, Arne was due to travel to Osaka for a world championships planning meeting. Ulla was going to stay at the temporary care accommodation. 'My trip to Japan had been preceded by a dreadful and decisive story at home. I was going to attend a meeting with the Swedish Sports Confederation. Ulla seemed calm. I thought it would be okay if I was away just for a couple of hours. Then suddenly she lost it. She went round and round in circles and then said to me: "Who are you?" In the same instant, she attacked me. She slapped me as hard as she could and scratched me, shouting in my face. I was afraid and bewildered. Then she collapsed as if she had fainted. She came to quite quickly and I saw no other option than to keep out of the way until she had calmed down, so I took my overcoat. Then she screamed: "You can't take that one. It's Arne's!" And then she collapsed again. When she came round, she didn't recall most of what had happened. I went for a walk around the neighbourhood to calm down. I took my mobile phone, turned it on and then it beeped: I had a voicemail. It was from the health centre in Danderyd. They were offering Ulla a place at Smedbygården in Åkersberga. It was a permanent place at a well-regarded home for people with dementia. I called them straight back. It was amazing that the offer of a place came just then. I made my decision the same day.'

In reality, it was a decision Arne had been preparing himself to take for a long time. It was a decision that would bring an end to the closeness that they had had for so many years. The love remained but their daily life together was over. 'I had lived with this thought for months and years. When the offer came it was like a godsend. I said that I would go there and talk to them at once.'

The next day, Håkan came to pick up Ulla and take her to the temporary sheltered accommodation. As soon as Arne returned from Osaka, she would be able to move in to Smedbygården. Ulla left her home in Enebyberg for the last time on March 22, 2006, the day before their forty-ninth wedding anniversary. 'When I saw Ulla and Håkan going down the steps before driving off, I knew it was the last time Ulla would be in the house. She would never return to live here. Then they got in the car and left and I thought: "She's leaving home now." It was incredibly painful. '

When Arne got back from Osaka, everything was agreed with Smedbygården. Together with Maria, his daughter, Arne went there to sort out Ulla's room. 'While we were standing there hanging up the curtains, Danderyd Hospital called. Ulla had disappeared from the sheltered accommodation.'

Ulla had disappeared before. They had once found her quite quickly in the library; another time she had managed to get further and was in the children's ward at the hospital. But this time they couldn't find her at the hospital. After half an hour she still hadn't been found. 'Another half hour passed and then my phone rang again. It wasn't the hospital. It was my neighbour in Enebyberg. He told me Ulla was at his place in his kitchen!'

Ulla had packed her things together and managed to get from the hospital to her house in Enebyberg, a distance of several kilometres. The neighbour had found her walking in the street outside her house. 'I'll never know how she managed it, how she found her way, or what thoughts must have been going through her head. It still hurts me deep in my soul when I think about her packing her bags and managing somehow to get home. Maybe she walked the whole way? And then she gets home and the doors are locked and she can't get in because she doesn't have a key. It's awful.'

They had planned to take Ulla straight to Smedbygården from the sheltered accommodation so she wouldn't get sad or upset by coming home in between. And then this happened. It was as if Ulla sensed what was going to happen.

Arne couldn't come and get her. It wouldn't work. Ulla would think that Arne had come to take her home. So it was Maria who went. She drove straight to Enebyberg. Ulla was happy to see her and went back with her in the car to Danderyd, thinking that she'd had a nice day out. 'The humour in all this shouldn't be underestimated. Back at the sheltered accommodation she was welcomed like a little heroine who had succeeded in escaping.'

On April 3, Ulla was driven out to her new home, Smedbygårdshemmet in Åkersberga, just twenty minutes by car from Enebyberg. She has lived there ever since.

THERE ARE EIGHT patients on each row at Smedbygårdshemmet. The entire place has seven rows, with a total of fifty-six inhabitants. Everyone has a big room and you can bring your own furniture and other things with you. There's a shared kitchen, a day-room and a TV room and then there's a large winter garden where everyone can meet. Everyday life is very plain, but it can't really be anything else.

Smedbygården's care approach is based on the notion that when memory disappears, it is the present moment that counts. You have to try and make the most of it as far as possible.

'It was awful to see Ulla immediately forgetting what had just happened. You just can't live together like that. She does much better at Smedbygården. Her short-term memory was zero. That's why she stopped reading; she didn't remember the page she had just read or even the previous sentence when she started the next one. We didn't have conversations either. There was none of the Ulla left that I knew to share memories with. What was important instead was whether she should have one or two lumps of sugar in her coffee. When she'd had one, she forgot she'd done it and so she had another and another and so on.

'Unfortunately Ulla has an aggressive component in her illness which not everyone has. There are Alzheimer's patients who, unlike Ulla, develop nice, docile, loyal behaviour. In contrast, Ulla has had many strong, aggressive outbursts. They've taken place when you least expect it and always completely unprovoked. She forgets them immediately, but for us relatives each hateful outburst remains. I notice that when I go to talk about them how indescribable it feels.'

Alzheimer's is sometimes called 'the relatives" disease'.

'It is an illness that you just can't handle in any way whatsoever. You can't reason with it. You can't put yourself in the sufferer's position either. It's awful to witness, especially when it is like half of your own being that's sick. And it's fatal: it's atrophy of the brain. It's a drawn out process. It usually takes ten to fifteen years from the start of the illness until your life is over.

'My Ulla has already gone. The illness consumed her and she disappeared. During the last twelve years she hasn't been the Ulla I know, except on fleeting occasions. It has been twelve very difficult years, and before that she had her deep depression. Sometimes I blame myself for all of it. I think that I could have done something different.

'I'm particularly taken by two accounts of Alzheimer's. One is Gösta Bohman's book about his wife. He was the Swedish finance minister in early 1990s. His wife also got Alzheimer's and went in to a home similar to Smedbygården. Bohman describes a different course of events than the ones I experienced, but at the same time our stories are very similar. Another account is Ulla Isaksson's novel *Boken om E* (*The Book About E*) which is about Erik Hjalmar Linder, a literary critic and an expert on Hjalmar Bergman. I've read everything by Bergman. He was a strange fellow, but a brilliant writer. And thanks to my interest in Bergman, I got to read a lot by Linder. He was a brilliant journalist, writer and lecturer. I didn't know that he suffered from Alzheimer's.'

Arne has been a successful doctor and lecturer. He has also been chairman of the Swedish Cancer Society. He has dedicated his whole life to helping others, teaching and lecturing. He has analysed and diagnosed illnesses and told people what they are suffering from, told them whether they will die now or tomorrow or be given the all-clear. Yet when it comes to the illness afflicting his wife, he has been utterly powerless. This has been hard to take.

'As a medical doctor, at least I have the advantage in that I understand more of what I read in the medical literature. Perhaps I also understand what is said in other texts in a different way, too. I remember a woman from a relatives-get-together at Smedbygården. With justified impatience she asked several questions: Why wasn't there any medicine? Why hasn't research come further than it has? Why is nothing happening?

'I tried to explain what I knew. I told her that actually, quite a lot has happened. In the 1950s, when I was studying medicine, the diagnosis of Alzheimer's was known but we didn't know much about it. Not what causes it, and not the nature of the changes to the brain. There weren't even clear criteria for diagnosing it back then. At that time distinction was only made between senile dementia – the dementia you get when you get old – and Alzheimer's, which was defined as "pre-senile dementia", in other words, a dementia that occurs at too early an age. Today we know much more. We know which changes occur in the brain and which diagnostic methods we should use to distinguish between different types of dementia, which is of course the first step towards prevention and treatment. Today we know that a precipitation of abnormal protein occurs around the brain cells which makes it harder for them to function and communicate, and in the worst of cases they cease functioning completely. And even that knowledge is a prerequisite for us to be able to find out how these changes occur and what we have to do to stop them or finally cure them. But many years of research remain.

'It's still not known how much of Alzheimer's is linked to genetic factors, whether it's hereditary or not. The illness hasn't been mapped out with genetics, only statistical data and that seems to indicate that children of an Alzheimer's patient are two or three times more at risk of developing the illness. It sounds like a big risk, but you should bear in mind that the actual absolute risk is very small. We don't know about Ulla's parents. They died so young. Of course, our children are worried that they will get it. But I think that they shouldn't worry about it unnecessarily. And you can count on preventative medication being available in some decades and maybe the illness will be treatable then, if not curable.'

WHILE ULLA'S ILLNESS created obvious difficulties when Arne took Ulla with him on larger social occasions, there were occasions when things could go well, even very late on in her illness. In December 2005, Arne was hosting an international gene doping seminar at the Karolinska Institutet with a dinner afterwards for fifty guests at Stadshuskällaren in Stockholm. Ulla sat at the table of honour next to a professor from California, a good friend of Arne who knew what the situation was.

'The whole dinner went well. It was the last big banquet I dared take her to. The last time we were out together for dinner among close friends was in May 2005, when the former European champion in high jump, Bengt Nilsson, and his wife Pia asked Ulla and I out to dinner together with Ulf Schmidt, the tennis pro who won the doubles at Wimbledon, and Ulf's wife

Karin, along with Hasse Rydén, a former top sprinter, and his wife Inga. Everyone knew about Ulla's disease which made me feel safe, which in turn made Ulla feel safe, so it was a successful evening.

'I think that a calm environment and people who are aware helps people suffering from Alzheimer's. She gets help to find her way in the here and now which is important. Like when we were invited to friends out on Blidö that summer. Erling Norrby, the researcher and former dean of the Karolinska Institute, and his wife invited us home to a wonderful summer lunch on Blidö together with the Lord Chamberlain Johan Fisherström and his wife. Everyone knew what was happening to Ulla and she was calm and happy.

'It's strange thinking back to that time. It was in March 2006 that Ulla went into care. We had the summer ahead of us and Ulla had been to Blidö every summer since 1949. I wondered how she would react but the summer passed without her so much as asking. Nothing about what we'd done together previous summers. Nothing about her beloved Blidö. Nothing. It is as if her old existence has been disconnected, as if it no longer exists.

'When you go through something like that as a relative, you also become a bit philosophical. Even if it is impossible to avoid growing old, you should strive to grow old in as gentle a way as possible. But this illness turns ageing into a living hell, and therefore it ought to be a field that medical researchers prioritise. The quality of life is severely worsened for many drawn out years. The course of the illness lasts for more than a decade and does not only affect the person who has it, but all their closest relatives.'

The question is left in the air. But it is painful to pose and difficult to answer. For a doctor it is a dilemma, for a close relative it can be impossible.

'Obviously I've thought along those lines, if it wouldn't have been better for Ulla to be allowed to die and avoid the last hellish years. Whether her life is meaningful for me or not, is not important. The point is I have great difficulty in believing that life as it is now is meaningful for Ulla. But we cannot know whether it is or not. The question remains and the discussion has been ongoing for as long as I can remember. Euthanasia? Active or passive? For or against? I once met a chap who was working at the IOC's headquarters. His mother-in-law also lived in Switzerland where they allow euthanasia. One day he told me that she was very sick and that the next morning she would receive help to end her life.

'This is a very important discussion. It has to be debated. But I have also witnessed first-hand how this problem is dealt with in practice within our healthcare system. The less rules the better, I think. Certainly, it is left up to the good judgement of the care workers to deal with the problems as they arise, but you have to trust that judgement.

'Towards the end of the 1950s I filled in at the paediatric ward at Karolinska University Hospital when a baby was born without the top of his cranium. We knew there was nothing we could do and that the child would get meningitis and encephalitis and die. This started a discussion of whether or not we should give him antibiotics. The idea was out of place in my view: antibiotics are supposed to be used to cure and such a severe defect can never be cured. This is an example of passively letting someone die as quickly as possible through withholding treatment.

'Another early experience which shaped my view occurred during the years I worked at Lovisa's Children's Hospital in the beginning of the 1960s. A Swedish family that was living abroad had come home for a summer holiday. Their son, who was about four, was not used to traffic driving on the left side of the road, as it was in Sweden back in those days. He was run down by a car and seriously injured. They put him on a respirator and all the resources at the emergency ward were used. But as it turned out, it was hopeless. He was brain dead, although the term had not been invented at the time. And there he lay, week after week on the respirator. Eventually, the father had to return to his job abroad. The mother remained grieving at her son's bedside. I could see how the mother sat fading away as the weeks passed. Finally, the boy died from pneumonia. I have often wondered what happened to the mother and father. How did they experience their time at the hospital? And how did they, in retrospect, see it? My own impression at least was that the mother aged ten years during those weeks.

'For my own part I think that the worst thing that could happen to me personally would be to have a stroke which rendered me severely handicapped. That would be devastating for me personally. My mobility, doing sport, have been my *raison d'être*. It would be distressing to think that I had to live without them for the last five to ten years of my life. Egotistically speaking, in such a situation I would welcome the chance to put an end to it all. But as concerns Ulla, I have not really been able to think that way. Ulla vanished for me a long time ago and the only thing that I am left with is the duty of going out to see her now and then. It hasn't just been inconvenient, but also often chaotic. The only reason to go there has been a short moment of recognition, and then not even that. Ulla has wandered out of my life and our relationship is gone. It's awful. Today she can neither talk, nor move. She is totally helpless.'

What is left is to get used to living alone, taking care of yourself, and perhaps adapting to a different life. Arne could leave the house now and move if he wanted to. It is cheaper to remain living where he is, but then there is the upkeep and the garden. Arne doesn't really need the house. He has, over the years, come closer to that decision. For a long time he didn't feel that Ulla had been gone long enough and that it would take a bit more time.

'In terms of my feelings there's no problem living there, but it will surely be an emotional upheaval to move. That is something I will have to deal with. And in any case I will have to move into something I really want. When I think about it, it will probably be something in one of the suburbs. I've never been one to live in the city. I can imagine some simple abode in the northern suburbs of Stockholm. Then again, I have the freedom of spending my summers on Blidö. We'll see.'

Postscript

ARNE WAS EIGHTY on Good Friday 2011. He retired fifteen years ago. He is hale and hearty, is very active, as he always has been. He takes the stairs instead of the lift. He likes to go cross-country skiing.

'Of course I have a little more aches and pains now than before, but I seem to have a good hereditary disposition to keep going in to old age. My father was physically strong and active. Although he died of a heart problem at seventy, he was fit to the end. And my mother was fit right up in to her nineties. I haven't had to worry about being in any danger zone. Besides, I've lived an interesting life. When I retired at the age of sixty-five I thought that I would cut down on my activities, but realised the importance of keeping something to stay active. I couldn't give up everything. I knew that it wasn't healthy.

'The big change that came about with my retirement was that I could control my own time. That was a great freedom. And even though I gave up my daily professional work, I still had my other assignments.'

It is only lately that he has cut down on his commitments. The first commitment that he asked to step down from was the Swedish Sports Confederation. That was in 1999. At the time he had been president for ten years and it took two more years until a suitable successor was found. The same year, in 2001, he also left his position at the Swedish Cancer Society having served as its president for three periods of three years each, the maximum time according to a rule that Arne himself had been involved in pushing through. He also left his post at court. He still had his commission within the IOC and WADA. He gave up his post at the IAAF when he became vice-president of WADA in 2007.

It has been a long life and there is a lot of work to look back upon. 'When I do that I really have no unfulfilled dreams. Each assignment has led to a steady stream of others, the whole time with a shared starting point, that being my medical qualifications and my interest in serving sport.

'Perhaps I've missed out on some things in life. For example, we haven't really had a large group of friends outside of those I met through my work. We're not the kind of people who like to be seen out and about all over the place, it's never really been our style. So I've chosen not to do that quite happily. I have, on the other hand, really valued my free time. I often stay on Blidö and have always ensured I've had more free time than many of my colleagues.

'There's nothing I regret. I've followed my desires and taken each possibility as it has come along. You don't regret very often the things you try. Perhaps you only regret the chances you didn't take. That's why I've always thought that I'll try. If there's not enough time or it does not suit me, it's just a case of not doing it any more. If there's anything I mourn it's for the talents that I don't have. The worst thing is that I am not musical. I can't sing. I've noticed from friends how much joy and fellowship there is from that. Some of my family on my father's side were musical, but I didn't inherit that. I've been sorry about that over the years.

'Ulla and I have largely been spared serious crises in our life together, at least until Ulla's illness. The biggest trauma that hit us was when Håkan's little girl Veronica turned out to have an incurable liver problem. I will never forget that day. I had a strange premonition as I recall. We were at the 1997 World Indoor Championships in Paris, and she can only have been ten days old or so when Håkan rang me. There couldn't be any problem with Veronica, could there?

'But there was. She was turning more and more yellow. The doctors told them it didn't look good and were of the opinion that her bile ducts were blocked. The bile wasn't emptying as it should. I understood then that it was serious. A poorly functioning bile duct system will ruin the liver. I had stood there myself and taught medical students about liver and bile duct diseases. It took several years of fighting until she was able to have a liver transplant. It was her uncle, her mother's half-brother Kalle, who donated a part of his liver. That happened in 2002. After that she's been fine.

'After all my years within healthcare, I know that this is the kind of thing that hits people. Both what has happened to Ulla and little Veronica are the kind of things that happen in life.'

WHEN HE LOOKS back at his life's work for sport, Arne thinks of a couple of things with particular satisfaction. One of them is the work he did on gender testing. 'Yes, it was a happy day the day I finally put an end to those humiliating gender tests. I had to work for fifteen years before the IOC grasped that the tests were unscientific and unethical and decided to cease using them. It was a decision that served as a guiding principle for the whole world of sport. It was enormously satisfying.'

And then there's his work against doping. 'Yes. Of course, it's the same thing there. I don't know what would have happened if I hadn't reacted. There's been an enormous change since I got involved in the work. I've carried a heavy load: first, in Sweden and then internationally. Today doping is a global political issue. We have a UNESCO convention against doping, and government representatives who sit at the same table as I do, discussing issues related to doping.

'We've had an American president who has taken up the problem of doping in his State of the Nation speech. It's been a fantastic journey since I began almost forty years ago. And most of all, nowadays people all around the world consciously recognise that doping is completely unacceptable. Doping is cheating, and doping is dangerous, both for the individual and for society in general. If there's anything that I shall be remembered for, it is this.'

At the same time the question how doping will be tackled in the future remains open. Will the 'doping industry' triumph over the 'doping police'? How will gene technology affect the work? Will pharmaceuticals, gene therapies and hormones be developed so that no method of analysis will spot them?

No, says Arne. 'There was a time when we were perhaps some fifteen years behind them, but now we're keeping up pretty much. Today we have methods of testing that are ready ahead of every big competition. We're at the same level as they are and in some aspects perhaps one step ahead of the doping industry. And we have permission to keep samples for eight years in order to conduct additional analysis on them should more sophisticated analytical methods be developed for chemicals that we could not analyse before.'

Perhaps Arne's work to combat doping can be described as a kind of pharmaceutical horserace. The pharmaceutical industry is one of the biggest industries in the world. And medical science is one of the most quickly advancing. It only takes about ten years to change the entire arsenal of medicine. One example of this is the anabolic steroids that broke through during the 1960s and 1970s. 'Even in 1974, we had a way of tracing these substances. Another example is testosterone. Because it is produced in the body, it was said that testosterone doping would be impossible to detect. But we simply measured the proportions between testosterone and another related hormone, epitestosterone, and the quotient told us if testosterone had been injected. Today, we have developed an even more reliable method which is called Isotope Ratio Mass Spectometry (IRMS) or "the carbon isotope method". It's based upon the fact that synthetic testosterone has a different proportion of carbon isotopes than what the body produces naturally.'

The big challenge for the future is perhaps gene technology and the risks this opens up for doping. 'When a laboratory in Pennsylvania reported that they had succeeded in getting muscle mass and skeletal structure to be strengthened by gene technology, I heard that athletes and coaches contacted them at once, asking to benefit from the new discovery. It's not just bad taste, it's also exceptionally scary. It can be extremely dangerous to undergo gene therapy. Up to now, gene therapy is an experimental practice which can only be allowed when treating very special illnesses and which requires rigorous supervision. In spite of this, unexpected deaths have occurred.'

As early as 2002, in his capacity as chairman of WADA's research committee, Arne arranged a conference at Cold Spring Harbour Laboratory in the United States, the same laboratory that first discovered the structure of DNA molecules. The conference brought together world-leading DNA researchers, representatives from the world of sport and legal experts. 'It turned out that we have the researchers on our side. They're anxious that gene therapy doesn't get into the hands of the wrong people, that could give rise to accidents and ruin the reputation of the science. We set up a working group to analyse how gene doping could be discovered and prevented in the future. The group is lead by Theodore Friedmann, the head of the Gene Therapy Center in La Jolla, California. When Friedmann was asked straight out about the possibilities to detect gene doping, he answered unequivocally: "There is," he said, "already a great possibility that scientists will discover a technique to trace gene doping. Anyone who thinks that it is possible to undergo gene doping without being caught will be surprised."

'A follow-up meeting was held in Stockholm in 2005, in collaboration with the Karolinska Institutet, WADA and the Swedish Sports Confederation, and another in St Petersburg in June 2008 together with the Russian anti-doping authorities. In 2010 two WADA-supported research teams independently reported findings which represent the first step towards the development of methods for the detection of gene doping.'

Voices are raised, sometimes from within the world of sport itself, against the sums of money that are put into tackling doping. Arne dismisses them categorically. 'There is an incredible amount of money circling about in sport. In the WADA accredited laboratories around the world, 250,000 tests are done annually. Each routine doping control costs about $500, which makes spending on tests about $125 million per year.

Postscript

'Yet just one ice hockey team in the NHL pays more money in wages to its players per year than we put into analysis work for anti-doping around the whole world. And there are individual athletes in sports like golf and tennis who have annual incomes that are several times larger than WADA's entire budget.

'Such facts in themselves are more than argument enough that more of the money that is circulating in the sports business should be freed up for the fight we're undertaking. It is vital in terms of the credibility of sport.'

Medicine has been Arne's profession, tackling doping his mission. But the world of sport is a part of the world as a whole, just a part of the complicated political context that continually influences it.

One example of politics' impact on sport are the recurring calls for sporting boycotts. Here Arne's basic position is crystal clear. 'I think that there are three areas that must be kept open between nations and regimes at any cost: science, sport and culture. I'm against boycotts on principal within these three fields. I believe that communication is the last thing that should cease if you get caught up in an international conflict. We have to keep a dialogue going with each other. We have to be able to keep the lines of communication open.'

Arne thinks that the risk is that there will be an unfortunate mixing of politics and sport.

'President Carter's boycott of the 1980 Moscow Olympics is a striking example. Today, few recall that the reason for the boycott was the Soviet invasion of Afghanistan. What good did that boycott do for Afghanistan? Those who suffered were the athletes who were denied the chance to compete in an Olympic Games. The same goes for the Eastern bloc's tit-for-tat boycott of the Los Angeles Games in 1984. They were two completely meaningless boycotts.

The only good that came out of it was that people began to discuss boycotts seriously.'

South Africa was more complicated. 'The principles of Swedish and international sport state that discrimination on the basis of gender, religion or race is not acceptable. The apartheid regime undertook a systematic programme of racial discrimination.

'And there were strong waves of support for the boycott of sport within South Africa. There was also the UN resolution which advocated a general isolation of South Africa, and stated that the sporting boycott was an important part of this. Within Swedish sport we made a decision in principle that still holds, to not take part in boycotts other than those sanctioned by the UN.'

But Arne notes that there are complications with a policy of isolation. He takes an example from science. Right in the middle of the South Africa boycott, the cardiac surgeon Christiaan Barnard undertook the first heart transplant in the world. 'A white man got a black man's heart, which led Sigge Ågren at the Swedish tabloid *Expressen* to run the following headline on the front page: "A black heart is just as red as a white one". It was a breakthrough that the whole world benefited from. And we would have been able to get more use out of Barnard's experiences at that time if the communications channels had been open. But I willingly admit that even South Africans believe that the sporting boycott benefited the South African people. I have heard this from people close to Mandela.'

Arne remembers how the discussions went ahead of the European Championships in Athens in 1969. Greece was in the hands of a military junta, and when the Swedish athletics association decided not to boycott, there was strong political pressure on the government to bring about a Swedish boycott. But Matts Carlgren, the president of the athletics association, received the following communication from prime minister Tage Erlander: 'I am convinced that the Swedish athletics association is competent to make the right decision.'

'Of course it was an excellent piece of political manoeuvring on Erlander's part, but at the same time it was an important demarcation for sport in our country, that sport can make its own decisions. I usually refer to it as "Erlander's Law".

'Of course, this doesn't mean that we are completely free to do as we please. We've always followed the foreign ministry's advice when it comes to travelling to places which are political trouble spots. Such consultation is intended to ensure the safety of athletes. In Greece in 1969, the association agreed to let the athletes themselves decide if they wanted to compete or not. And when Anders Gärderud and others elected to remain in Sweden, their decision was respected.'

It is absurd that sport should be used as a political weapon when other sectors of society retain connections. 'Sport's officials take care of sport and the politics of sport, not world politics. That is something politicians should take responsibility for. There have been many cases where sporting boycotts might have been used as a political tool: Israel, Iran, Iraq, Sri Lanka, Afghanistan, Soviet Union, North Korea, Burma … the list goes on. If it had been used each time, sport would have ceased to be an international bridge-builder. Instead, the most controversial countries are still part of the IOC and so involved in international sport.

'I believe that the political significance of sport as a bridge-builder is stronger now than it has ever been. Just think of when North and South Korea marched in under the same flag for the first time at the opening of the Summer Olympics in Sydney. Politicians haven't achieved this, despite enormous efforts and negotiations. It was Samaranch who made it happen. It was his diplomatic dexterity that gave results. This is surely a signal to the politicians about how the people on the Korean peninsula really want things.'

AHEAD OF THE 2008 Olympics in Beijing, there was again talk of a boycott, due to unease over the situation in Tibet, and then when the Buddhist monks demonstrated in Rangoon in Burma. Many called for the boycott of China because of the offences against human rights that are carried out within that country's borders. 'I was bombarded with stacks of letters, both from Sweden and abroad, saying that we were wrong to award the Olympic Games to Beijing, to a country that does not respect human rights. But these calls for a boycott come from people who are not close to sport, and cannot understand that sport is something completely different to politics.'

Instead, Arne insists that sport can actually open up a dialogue. During his many preparatory trips to Beijing ahead of the Games, he has seen for himself how the Chinese have changed their attitude. 'They've quite simply been forced to open up to greater international scrutiny, to a degree that they have never had to before. In the run-up to the Olympics, the visiting international delegations have taken over, demanding to know things that China would never have accepted before. Sometimes I wonder if China really was aware how all-encompassing the need to be open really was when they applied for the Olympics. Many of the international demands have probably come as a shock to the Chinese. I have understood from friends in China that some people appreciate the international inspection that the country was going through. Others don't.

'Personally, I think this close examination was good for China and the rest of the world, and that it continues to be so. We get to know each other and better understand one another. And I think that precisely that aspect should be taken into consideration if we're talking about sport's role in politics. When I first visited China in 1978, it was my involvement in sport that got me admitted to the country, even though I wanted to study their medical training programme. And we would never dream of breaking off the scientific contacts with China. It would be absurd. I know myself just how much there is to discover from each other because we've had a stream of Chinese doctoral students at the Karolinska Institutet since back when I was pro-vice-chancellor.'

The Olympic Games in Beijing became a great success, both for the Olympic movement and for the hosts. Many speculations about doping and other worries about political manifestations, security problems and poor environment proved to be unfounded. Doping never became a big issue during Games time. The sole press conference on that matter that Arne had to organise related to the successful identification by the IAAF of a handful of top Russian distance runners who had manipulated their urine samples at doping controls conducted well before Games time. Those athletes were barred from taking part at the Games. 'But for the first time we made use of a rule which allows for follow-up analysis of samples with methods that were not available at the time of the Games. Thus, we started in February 2009 to analyse a large number of samples for the new generation of EPO (CERA), as well as for insulin, since validated methods of testing for those substances had not been developed until after the host city contract was signed. In June it was confirmed that five athletes tested positive for CERA, raising the number of positive dope tests during the Games to fourteen. One of the five athletes found with CERA was a gold medallist.'

As the Games came closer, some visa problems were reported, but no incidents related to security or politics. However, the increasingly intense media reports about Beijing's unhealthy smog were troublesome, though they proved to be nothing but speculation.

'In March 2008, we issued a press release from the IOC medical commission with information about the measures that were being undertaken by the Chinese authorities and which suggested that the environmental conditions for athletes and visitors at the Beijing Games would be fully acceptable and safe. Yet, the propaganda around Beijing's air conditions continued, fuelled by some uninformed statements by top athletes. And when some athletes arrived in Beijing wearing masks to protect them from the air, for good reason the Chinese took offence. It turned out that the air quality throughout the Games was more than acceptable. This was confirmed both by hourly reports that we received from strategically positioned measurement stations, and by satellite studies that had been conducted by NASA and were released in December 2008.'

Indeed, the NASA report concluded that the measures that the Beijing authorities had undertaken in order to clean up the air were unexpectedly successful and a good example what could be done for the environment. Some of those measures will be of permanent benefit for the Beijing population, such as the moving of dirty factories out of the city, and a smoking ban in public places.

Tobacco smoking is a major threat to public health globally. In China, it is of exceptional importance. One-third of the world's smokers live in China. About sixty to seventy per cent of Chinese men between thirty and sixty years of age are smokers. And there is evidence that smoking is becoming increasingly common among young women. To reduce tobacco smoking is, therefore, of particular importance for the long-term health of the Chinese people.

The decision by China's authorities to maintain after the Games some of the restrictions on the use of private cars can also be expected to be a significant factor promoting health. 'I do not believe that the environmental aspects would have been on the political agenda in China to the extent that they were had the Olympic Games not been awarded to Beijing. The matter has received the attention of the World Health Organisation, and we now have developed a joint project with the Beijing Municipal Health Bureau, the Organising Committee of the Games, the IOC medical commission and WHO entitled "The health legacy of the Beijing Olympic Games". The report, published by WHO in May 2010, is intended to serve as a basis for follow-up studies. As a scientist I should be careful in not being biased, but I have to confess that it would be wonderful if it could be shown that the decision to stage the Olympic Games in Beijing resulted in long-term improvement of the health of its inhabitants.'

A dream scenario for the IOC Medical Committee chairman and a wonderful example of the important role that the Olympic Games can play.

INDEX

Index